Is Enough Being Done to Protect Athletes from Concussions?

Christine Wilcox

INCONTROVERSY

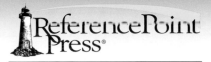

ReferencePoint
Press®

San Diego, CA

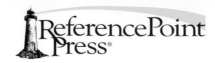

© 2015 ReferencePoint Press, Inc.
Printed in the United States

For more information, contact:
ReferencePoint Press, Inc.
PO Box 27779
San Diego, CA 92198
www.ReferencePointPress.com

LIBRARY OF CONGRESS CATALOGING-IN-PUBLICATION DATA

Wilcox, Christine.
   Is enough being done to protect athletes from concussions? / by Christine Wilcox.
      pages cm. -- (In controversy)
   Includes bibliographical references and index.
      ISBN 978-1-60152-754-7 (hardback) -- ISBN 1-60152-754-3 (hardback) 1. Brain--Concussion--Prevention. 2. Soccer injuries--Prevention. 3. Sports injuries--Prevention. 4. High school athletes--Wounds and injuries--Prevention. 5. College athletes--Wounds and injuries--Prevention. I. Title.
   RC394.C7W55   2015
   617.1'027--dc23
                                                                          2014024366

Contents

Foreword   4

Introduction
Concussions Damage the Brain   6

Chapter One
What Are the Origins of the Concussion Controversy
in Sports?   11

Chapter Two
How Dangerous Are Concussions?   26

Chapter Three
Are Adult Leagues Doing Enough to Protect Players?   40

Chapter Four
Are Schools and Youth Leagues Doing Enough to
Protect Kids?   54

Chapter Five
Who Is to Blame for Concussion Risks to Athletes?   67

Source Notes   80

Related Organizations and Websites   85

Additional Reading   88

Index   91

Picture Credits   95

About the Author   96

Foreword

In 2008, as the US economy and economies worldwide were falling into the worst recession since the Great Depression, most Americans had difficulty comprehending the complexity, magnitude, and scope of what was happening. As is often the case with a complex, controversial issue such as this historic global economic recession, looking at the problem as a whole can be overwhelming and often does not lead to understanding. One way to better comprehend such a large issue or event is to break it into smaller parts. The intricacies of global economic recession may be difficult to understand, but one can gain insight by instead beginning with an individual contributing factor, such as the real estate market. When examined through a narrower lens, complex issues become clearer and easier to evaluate.

This is the idea behind ReferencePoint Press's *In Controversy* series. The series examines the complex, controversial issues of the day by breaking them into smaller pieces. Rather than looking at the stem cell research debate as a whole, a title would examine an important aspect of the debate such as *Is Stem Cell Research Necessary?* or *Is Embryonic Stem Cell Research Ethical?* By studying the central issues of the debate individually, researchers gain a more solid and focused understanding of the topic as a whole.

Each book in the series provides a clear, insightful discussion of the issues, integrating facts and a variety of contrasting opinions for a solid, balanced perspective. Personal accounts and direct quotes from academic and professional experts, advocacy groups, politicians, and others enhance the narrative. Sidebars add depth to the discussion by expanding on important ideas and events. For quick reference, a list of key facts concludes every chapter. Source notes, an annotated organizations list, bibliography, and index provide student researchers with additional tools for papers and class discussion.

The *In Controversy* series also challenges students to think critically about issues, to improve their problem-solving skills, and to sharpen their ability to form educated opinions. As President Barack Obama stated in a March 2009 speech, success in the twenty-first century will not be measurable merely by students' ability to "fill in a bubble on a test but whether they possess 21st century skills like problem-solving and critical thinking and entrepreneurship and creativity." Those who possess these skills will have a strong foundation for whatever lies ahead.

No one can know for certain what sort of world awaits today's students. What we can assume, however, is that those who are inquisitive about a wide range of issues; open-minded to divergent views; aware of bias and opinion; and able to reason, reflect, and reconsider will be best prepared for the future. As the international development organization Oxfam notes, "Today's young people will grow up to be the citizens of the future: but what that future holds for them is uncertain. We can be quite confident, however, that they will be faced with decisions about a wide range of issues on which people have differing, contradictory views. If they are to develop as global citizens all young people should have the opportunity to engage with these controversial issues."

In Controversy helps today's students better prepare for tomorrow. An understanding of the complex issues that drive our world and the ability to think critically about them are essential components of contributing, competing, and succeeding in the twenty-first century.

Concussions Damage the Brain

Pittsburgh Steelers center Michael "Iron Mike" Webster was one of the most respected and admired football players of all time. He and Terry Bradshaw led the Steelers to four Super Bowl victories between 1974 and 1980. Webster was the team's leader; he was smart and tough, and he prided himself on being able to play through any injury. He also had a reputation for using his head as a battering ram, smashing it into the defensive line on every play. Former New York Giants linebacker Harry Carson said the only way to neutralize Webster was to hit him in the face. "That's what we were taught," Carson said, "to hit a guy right in the face so hard that they're dazed and stunned."[1] Webster even developed a thick layer of scar tissue on his forehead from hitting and being hit in the same spot over and over. According to former Steelers running back Merril Hoge, Webster was "the epitome of the NFL. Nobody was as tough as that dude. Nobody."[2]

Despite his ferocity on the field, Webster was known to be an intelligent, thoughtful, easygoing man. But after his retirement, he began to change. He became short-tempered, distracted, and forgetful. He began to behave erratically—leaving home for weeks at a time and spending all his money on irresponsible investments until he had bankrupted his family. His wife divorced him, and afterward he drifted from place to place, often sleeping in bus stations. He was in constant pain, and he found it impossible to focus without massive doses of Ritalin, a drug that improves concentration. Soon he was convinced that football had destroyed his brain, and he often threatened to quit the Hall of Fame in protest of the NFL's treatment of him and other retired players.

Before his death of a heart attack in 2002, Webster began to show signs of dementia. He would lose his way on short trips to the corner store and once mistook his open oven door for a urinal. His sons took care of him in the last years of his life. He was in so much mental and physical pain that he would beg to be shocked to unconsciousness with a Taser. It was the only way he could sleep.

Webster had chronic traumatic encephalopathy (CTE), a neurodegenerative disease caused by repetitive brain injury. CTE is only revealed during autopsy; Webster's brain showed the distinctive pattern of damage typical of the disease. Since his death CTE has been found in the brains of nearly fifty deceased NFL players—many of whom were so devastated by the disease during life that they committed suicide. Thousands of other former players

After retiring from football, Pittsburgh Steelers center Mike Webster (wearing number 52) suffered severe health problems that were later determined to be the result of the multiple head injuries he received during his career.

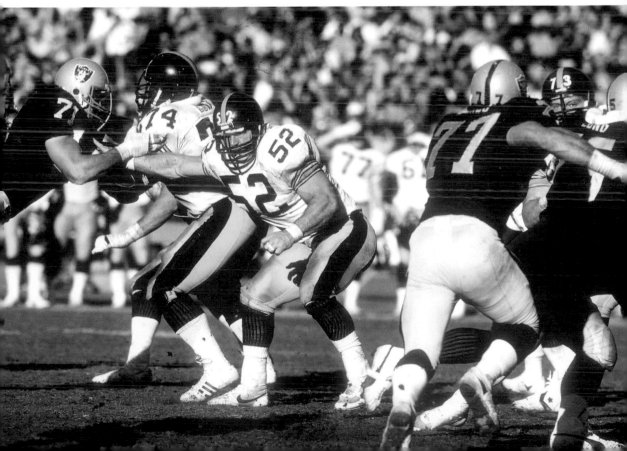

are suffering from symptoms of CTE or other concussion-related brain disorders, and they have joined together to sue the NFL. They claim that the NFL deliberately misled them about the long-term effects of concussions, which can include neurodegenerative diseases such as amyotrophic lateral sclerosis (ALS), Parkinson's disease, and early onset Alzheimer's disease.

Educating the Public

The controversy in the NFL has served to educate the public about the dangers of concussions. Until very recently many people considered a concussion to be a minor injury. An athlete who was woozy after being hit on the head was described as getting "dinged" or "getting his bell rung," and a player's ability to recover from a concussion was thought to be a sign of toughness—as if it were something in that player's control. For instance, in 1994 Dr. Elliot Pellman, chair of the NFL's Mild Traumatic Brain Injury (MTBI) Committee, said, "Concussions are part of the profession, an occupational risk."[3] He claimed that veteran football players recover from concussions "more quickly than rookies. They can unscramble their brains a little faster, maybe because they're not afraid after being dinged."[4] Fifteen years later the NFL still had not changed its position; in 2009 its brain injury committee published a study in the medical journal *Neurosurgery* that concluded that concussions in professional football did not cause brain damage.

This attitude has since been proved wrong. Concussions are serious brain injuries that if not treated correctly can cause permanent brain damage, neurodegenerative diseases, or death. The Centers for Disease Control and Prevention estimates that 3.8 million or more sports-related concussions occur in the United States each year. About 10 percent of concussion sufferers develop post-concussion syndrome—a condition that causes searing headaches, confusion, problems with thinking, and emotional instability. The odds of suffering from post-concussion syndrome go up if the brain is not allowed to heal, causing the condition to linger for months or even years and devastating the lives of those who suffer from it. In young people

" Concussions are part of the profession, an occupational risk."[3]

— Dr. Elliot Pellman, former chair of the NFL's MTBI Committee.

the effects of concussions and post-concussion syndrome are even more pronounced and can even lead to sudden death.

Sports Are Changing

After years of denial, the NFL finally admitted that concussions in football can lead to brain damage. In 2009 NFL spokesperson Greg Aiello said, "It's quite obvious from the medical research that's been done that concussions can lead to long-term problems."[5] The league began to take steps to reduce the incidence of sports concussions and make the game safer for its players. Concussion analysis tools were improved, and teams began to take a baseline reading of players' cognitive functions before each season. Contact in practice was reduced. Head hits were outlawed, and rules were changed to eliminate the most dangerous plays. Other sports leagues, including college and youth leagues, followed the NFL's lead, adopting many of the NFL's concussion policies and modifying their own rules of play.

"It's quite obvious from the medical research that's been done that concussions can lead to long-term problems."[5]

— Greg Aiello, NFL spokesperson.

Today many people are protesting these changes, claiming that the sports they love are becoming watered down and boring. Others want to see many more changes made, such as eliminating the kickoff in football and ending body checking in ice hockey. Still others have decided that contact sports are simply too dangerous—especially for children. Parents worry that the games they loved as children might be putting their own children's brains at risk, and they have begun to pull their kids out of sports. Between 2011 and 2013 enrollment in youth football dropped about 10 percent.

Because of concerns about sports concussions, many predict that contact sports will soon disappear from American life—or will be changed so much that they will be unrecognizable. Others believe that sports like football are so intertwined with American culture that they will never disappear. One thing is certain—only by fully understanding the issues can society hope to keep its athletes safe from the devastating effects of sports concussions.

Facts

- According to the Brain Research Institute, a traumatic brain injury such as concussion occurs every fifteen seconds.

- The University of Pittsburgh Medical Center estimates that at least 10 percent of all contact sports athletes sustain concussions yearly.

- A study published in the *Clinical Journal of Sports Medicine* found that only 47 percent of high school football players report their concussions.

CHAPTER ONE

What Are the Origins of the Concussion Controversy in Sports?

The story of how concussions were finally taken seriously in the sports community is a long and complex one. Since concussions occur most frequently in contact sports, most of the controversy centered on the NFL—a multibillion dollar industry that had the most to lose by the revelation that concussions cause brain damage. Critics have accused the NFL of spending years in denial about the dangers of concussions. Some even believe NFL officials purposely withheld information about those dangers from players and the public. According to ex-professional wrestler Chris Nowinski, codirector of Boston University's Center for the Study of Traumatic Encephalopathy, "The concussion issue was covered up, kept from the American people for—I mean, let's be honest—decades longer than it

" The concussion issue was covered up, kept from the American people for—I mean, let's be honest—decades longer than it should have been."6

— Former professional wrestler Chris Nowinski, codirector of the Center for the Study of Traumatic Encephalopathy.

should have been."[6] NFL players were not the only ones affected; since most other professional sports leagues cannot fund their own concussion research, they often looked to the NFL for best practices about concussions—and their players suffered for it. According to Nowinski, countless athletes—both adults and children—have been unnecessarily injured over the past two decades because they followed NFL concussion policies.

Punch-Drunk Syndrome

CTE is not a new disease. It was first discovered in professional boxers in 1928 by pathologist Harrison Stanford Martland. At that time it was called punch-drunk syndrome or dementia pugilistica, which means "boxer's dementia." The condition is caused by repeated concussions—in this case, punches to the head—and is characterized by memory loss and the early onset of dementia. Martland estimated that almost half of all retired pro boxers had the condition. In 1957 neurologist MacDonald Critchley published a study that indicated that dementia pugilistica was progressive, advancing steadily even after a boxer stops fighting. Critchley also found that "there may be mood swings, intense irritability, and sometimes truculence leading to uninhibited violent behavior" and that "sometimes there is depression with a paranoid colouring."[7]

By 1972 it was widely accepted in the medical community that dementia pugilistica was caused by repeated brain trauma. However, no one in the boxing world wanted to hear that the essence of the sport caused brain damage. The boxing establishment argued that there was no way to prove it was boxing, rather than drug use or an unknown disease, that caused the brain atrophy and enlarged ventricles (chambers that contain cerebrospinal fluid) that are characteristic of dementia pugilistica. Besides, other than outlawing blows to the head, there was little that could be done to protect boxers except to inform them of the risks. According to neurologist Ira Casson, who examined the CAT scans of several boxers—including ex-heavyweight champion Muhammad Ali—for an article in *Sports Illustrated* in 1983, "A boxer ought to know what he's getting into if he wants to go on and be a champion. He should know what he may be sacrificing. A doctor has to

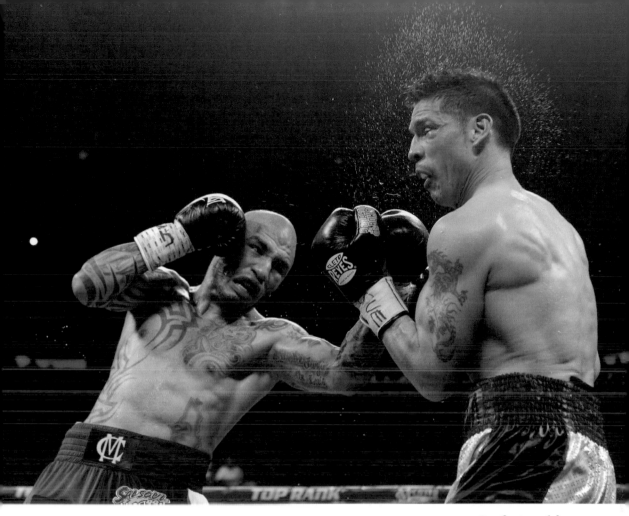

tell the boxer if he thinks the fighter should stop, but in the end it's not really a medical decision."[8]

Baseline Testing

By 1990 nearly everyone in sports was familiar with punch-drunk syndrome in boxers. However, almost no one outside of the medical community made the connection between concussions sustained in the boxing ring and those sustained in other contact sports, like football and ice hockey. At the time, there was hardly any research on sports concussions, and the guidelines for how long an athlete should rest after sustaining a concussion were not backed up by any scientific studies.

Neurosurgeon Joseph Maroon, who volunteered as a consul-

Professional boxers such as Puerto Rico's Miguel Cotto and Argentina's Sergio Martinez (right) risk a form of dementia known as "punch-drunk syndrome" that is caused by repeated blows to the head.

tant to the Pittsburgh Steelers, set out to change this in 1991. He and neuropsychologist Mark Lovell instituted a program of baseline neurological testing before the season began. Then, if a player became disoriented after a hit, he would take another test, right on the sidelines, and its results would be compared to the baseline. This would show with a fair amount of accuracy if the player had a concussion and how severe it was.

One of the players who participated in baseline testing was Merril Hoge. Hoge had been concussed many times, but like most athletes at the time, he did not realize that dizziness, or "seeing stars," was a sign of a concussion or that the effects of concussions tended to be cumulative. Then in 1994 Hoge left the Steelers and joined the Chicago Bears, where he suffered two serious concussions in the first six weeks of the season. After the second, Hoge's short-term memory was shot—he could not even remember the name of his two-year-old daughter. He returned to Pittsburgh, hoping that Maroon and Lovell could tell him why he was not getting any better.

Hoge was tested again, and the doctors were shocked by the results. Compared to his baseline tests, Hoge's scores had dropped by half. Maroon called Hoge into his office and said, "You do this to your brain again, I can't help you. Whatever happens, it's done, it's final, it's finished. If you drool or you can't speak or you can't function, I can't do anything about that."[9] Hoge got the message—he was one hit away from permanent brain damage. At twenty-nine years old, Hoge retired from the NFL.

The Season of the Concussion

Hoge was just one of many high-profile players who sustained serious concussions in 1994, which *League of Denial* authors Mark Fainaru-Wada and Steve Fainaru dubbed the "Season of the Concussion."[10] Another was Dallas Cowboys quarterback Troy Aikman, who took a knee to the head during the NFC Championship game on January 23, 1994. Later that night, his agent, Leigh Steinberg, visited him in the hospital. Steinberg told *Frontline* that not only did Aikman have no memory of playing the game, but his short-term memory was so impaired that he could not retain information for more than a few minutes. Aikman asked Steinberg over and over again if they had won the game. Steinberg was shaken by Aikman's condition: "It terrified me to see how tender the bond was between sentient consciousness and potential dementia and confusion."[11]

The Mild Traumatic Brain Injury Committee

In response to the growing concern about concussions, in 1994 NFL commissioner Paul Tagliabue created the Mild Traumatic Brain Injury (MTBI) Committee. The committee was formed to conduct research into the effects of concussions on NFL players and, if they were indeed found to be a problem, to explore ways to reduce their incidence. However, it soon became clear that even though Tagliabue created the committee, he did not believe concussions were an issue. He asserted again and again that the overall rate of concussions in the NFL was quite low. He also only appointed three brain specialists to the committee. The rest of the members were all NFL insiders—team doctors, trainers, and equipment managers. And the chair of the committee was rheumatologist Elliot Pellman. Pellman was the team doctor for the Jets and Tagliabue's personal physician, and he had a reputation for sending concussed players back on the field. Pellman had never published a paper on concussions. In fact, according to neurophysiologist Bill Barr, who also consulted with the Jets, Pellman often told coaches and trainers that no research existed on concussions and the MTBI Committee was starting from scratch. "I had been trained in evaluating MTBI, and I knew the literature," Barr said. "But he acted like nothing had ever been published on this before 1995."[12]

A Devastating Disease

Over the next several years, research on concussions progressed slowly. Then in 2002 a young neuropathologist named Bennet Omalu autopsied the brain of former Pittsburgh Steelers center Mike Webster. Omalu did so on a hunch. He noted that Webster's medical history said he was suffering from post-concussion syndrome—a condition associated with symptoms such as headaches, cognitive difficulties, and irritability. Even though Webster died of

Five Concussions a Game

In 1994 Leigh Steinberg was agent to almost every quarterback in the NFL. After seeing how profoundly a concussion affected Troy Aikman, he set up informational seminars to educate the players. One of the attendees was San Francisco 49ers linebacker Gary Plummer. When a presenter described Grade 1 concussion symptoms as being slightly disoriented and "seeing stars," Plummer interrupted him. "If I didn't have five of your so-called Grade 1 concussions a game," he said, "I was basically inactive. And by the way, there are some plays when you get *two* of those on the same play. You try putting your forehead underneath a 330-pound offensive guard and then get off of him to take on a 220-pound running back. Trust me, you're going to see stars." Plummer estimated that, going by the neurologists' guidelines, he had had more than 750 concussions in his career.

Years later, after seeing the devastation concussions had inflicted on his fellow players, Plummer had a change of heart. "It's still remarkable to think how uneducated I was," he said in 2013. "I'd love to go back and say, 'I'm sorry, I was a moron.' But that was the attitude at the time."

Quoted in Mark Fainaru-Wada and Steve Fainaru, *League of Denial*. New York: Crown, 2013, Kindle edition.

heart failure, Omalu wondered if a neurodegenerative disease like Alzheimer's had contributed to his death.

What Omalu saw in Webster's brain tissue shocked him. Webster's brain looked normal to the naked eye, but microscopic examination revealed that it was clogged with tangles of a tar-like protein called tau. The tangles were a sign of Alzheimer's, but the brain had no other hallmarks of the disease. Omalu showed the samples to his mentor, Dr. Ronald Hamilton, who immediately asked Omalu if the subject had been a boxer. The tangles of tau looked like dementia pugilistica—yet the brain itself was not atrophied and the ventricles were not enlarged.

Omalu had found something no one had ever seen before: a strain of dementia pugilistica caused by inadvertent concussions rather than deliberate blows to the head. It was something completely new. He and Hamilton decided to call it chronic traumatic encephalopathy.

Later Omalu and Hamilton showed their discoveries to Maroon with the hope that he would assist them with a research study. After Maroon had examined the slides, he asked Omalu, "Do you understand the impact of what you're doing?" When Omalu, a Nigerian who knew nothing about American football, asked him what he meant, Maroon said, "If only 10 percent of mothers in America begin to conceive of football as a dangerous game, that is the end of football."[13]

The *Journal of No NFL Concussions*

By the time that Omalu made his discovery, the NFL's MTBI Committee was publishing its own research in the medical journal *Neurosurgery*, which was edited by neurosurgeon Michael Apuzzo, a consultant to the New York Giants. Like all respected scientific journals, *Neurosurgery* used the peer review process, which means that before research is published, its validity is reviewed by other experts in the field. The process is intended to prevent research of questionable credibility from becoming part of the accepted body of scientific knowledge. If most peer reviewers reject an article, so does the journal.

Most of the MTBI Committee's articles were rejected by *Neurosurgery*'s peer reviewers. The articles all made the argument that concussions in football are minor injuries with no lasting effects, and that nearly all professional football players recover quickly and completely—assertions that were not backed up by reliable data and that contradicted the latest research in the field. However, instead of rejecting the articles, Apuzzo published them along

Safe to Return to Play?

Perhaps the most damaging statement in the MTBI Committee's published research was in their seventh paper, which claimed in 2005 that returning to a game after a concussion posed no significant risk. In the conclusion, the authors stated that "it might be safe for college/high school football players to be cleared to return to play on the same day as their injury." There was no evidence to back up this claim—young players had not even been studied. Yet because it appeared in *Neurosurgery*, it became part of accepted scientific knowledge.

Not only did the statement mislead youth football leagues about the seriousness of concussions, it misled participants of sports that modeled their concussion guidelines on the NFL's. In 2007 Dr. Gerard Malanga, director of the New Jersey Sports Medicine Institute and doctor to several local sports teams, said that parents, coaches, and players frequently "reference back to that article. It creates confusion when there's increasing clarity on the subject. They say what I tell them about it not being safe to go back in the same game is totally wrong, and they're backed by the NFL. So they go to a doctor who tells them what they want to hear."

Elliot J. Pellman et al., "Concussion in Professional Football: Players Returning to the Same Game—Part 7," *Neurosurgery*, January 2005, p. 89.

Quoted in Alan Schwarz, "NFL Study Authors Dispute Concussion Finding," *New York Times*, June 10, 2007. www.nytimes.com.

with the peer reviewers' commentaries. As one reviewer, Dr. Kevin Guskiewicz, said, "We were, like, 'Who reads the commentaries?' It's a published paper. It became the gospel."[14]

Guskiewicz and the other reviewers began to suspect that the sole purpose of the MTBI Committee was to establish a body of scientific research that could be called on to defend the NFL in the case of a lawsuit. After a while, they refused to review the papers, but Apuzzo simply found other peer reviewers. In all, *Neurosurgery* published sixteen of the MTBI Committee's research papers. Some researchers began to refer to the publication as the *Journal of No NFL Concussions*.

While *Neurosurgery* may have accepted subpar research from the MTBI Committee, it did not publish only one point of view. In 2005 Omalu published his research on Mike Webster's brain in *Neurosurgery*. The MTBI Committee immediately demanded that the paper be retracted—an extremely serious action reserved for charges of fraud or plagiarism. However, the committee's objections to Omalu's claims—that Webster had a variant of dementia pugilistica caused by playing football—were based on a misunderstanding of the science. Omalu and his coauthors wrote a response that addressed the committee's misconceptions, and Omalu's paper stood. It was now established in the medical literature that a former NFL player, who had suffered for years from cognitive and emotional problems, was found to have extensive brain damage caused by concussions.

Deaths Related to CTE

Webster's was the first in a long line of deaths that were related to CTE. In 2004 former Pittsburgh Steeler Justin Strzelczyk was suffering from extreme paranoia when he was killed in a police chase, slamming his car into a tanker truck at 140 miles per hour (225 kph) and dying in the explosion. The next year former Steeler Terry Long committed suicide by drinking antifreeze. In 2006 former Philadelphia Eagles defensive lineman Andre Waters shot himself in the head. Each of these men had CTE—which had devastated their lives in the years before their deaths. None of them were older than forty-five, and all of them were former linemen—tough players who took pride in playing through concussions. When Waters was asked in 1994 how he dealt with the fifteen or more concussions he had suffered so far in the NFL, he said, "In most cases, nobody knew it but me. I just wouldn't say anything. I'd sniff some smelling salts, then go back out there."[15]

CTE was proving to be not just a problem for football players. Several professional wrestlers had also been found to have the disease after death—the most notable being Chris Benoit. In 2007 Benoit drugged and murdered his wife and seven-year-old son and then hanged himself. His motives were unclear until former wrestler and concussion advocate Chris Nowinski contacted Benoit's father and suggested that Benoit may have been suffering from CTE. Nowinski had been working with Omalu to raise awareness about concussions, and Michael Benoit agreed to allow Omalu to examine his son's brain. An autopsy revealed that every section of Benoit's brain was clogged with tangles of tau protein. His brain resembled that of an eighty-five-year-old Alzheimer's patient.

Concussion Advocacy

Nowinski, a graduate of Harvard University, had become interested in the effects of concussions after sustaining several of them as a professional wrestler. Even though wrestling matches were scripted, the wrestlers' physical moves were real—they routinely

Chris Nowinski (third from left), a former wrestler who founded an organization devoted to raising awareness about the effects of sports concussions, looks on as a trio of doctors examine the brain of a deceased former football player.

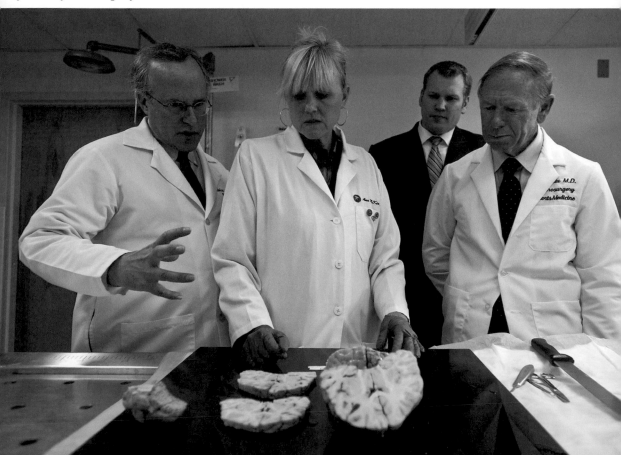

kicked each other in the head, hit each other with folding chairs, and threw each other to the ground. Nowinski suffered a series of concussions in 2003 that left him with severe headaches, poor short-term recall, and debilitating depression—which was later identified as post-concussion syndrome. None of his doctors could explain why he was not getting better, and eventually he gave up wrestling and began to research concussions on his own. In 2007 he published *Head Games*, which was made into an award-winning documentary about the risks of sports concussions.

Nowinski's research put him in contact with Omalu, with whom he founded the Sports Legacy Institute—a research institute devoted to raising awareness about sports concussions and CTE. Nowinski, who had no medical training, took over the role of "brain chaser"—if a death was reported that he suspected was caused by CTE, he would contact the family and request that they allow the institute to study their loved one's brain. Most families were cooperative. Like Chris Benoit's father, they wanted answers.

Nowinski had a knack for advocacy. In his opinion, the scientific method was far too slow—it could take years to publish new research and even longer for that information to filter down to the public. Nowinski wanted the public to know about CTE as soon as possible. He formed an alliance with *New York Times* sports writer Alan Schwarz, who wrote a feature story about Waters's suicide and went on to cover the concussion controversy in depth. Schwarz brought the controversy to the forefront of the public's awareness. Nowinski also decided that the Sports Legacy Institute should move to Boston University, where it would have more credibility and resources.

Nowinski and Omalu both had big personalities, and there was often conflict between them. They parted ways before the move to Boston, and Omalu eventually founded the Brain Injury Research Institute. Nowinski asked neuropathologist Ann McKee to join the Sports Legacy Institute, which expanded to form the Center for the Study of Traumatic Encephalopathy. McKee, an engaging speaker, was not only fascinated by tau proteins, she was a die-hard Green Bay Packers fan. She was the perfect person to take Omalu's place.

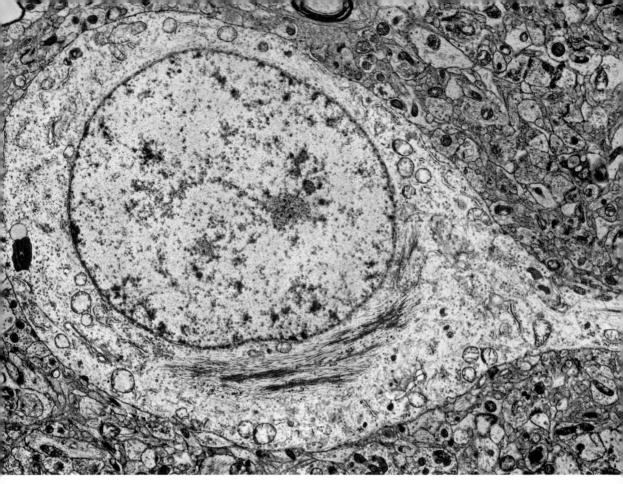

The red area in this microscopic image of a brain cell is a tangle of tau protein, a telltale sign of Alzheimer's disease and other brain disorders.

Football Itself May Cause CTE

One of the first brains that McKee examined belonged to Tom McHale, a former offensive guard for the Miami Dolphins who died in May 2008 of an accidental drug overdose. He was forty-five years old. After nine years in the NFL, McHale—who had graduated from Cornell University and had a warm, charismatic personally—gradually became so depressed that he lost interest in everything. Because he had no history of concussions, his wife thought the donation would be useful as an example of a healthy brain. She was wrong. McHale's brain was riddled with tau. McKee later told *Frontline*, "It was about as bad as you get. . . . There were what we call neurofibrillary tangles everywhere. They were throughout his hippocampus. They were throughout his frontal lobe. I had never seen anything like it in a person so young."[16] And the fact that

McHale had never had a concussion supported a theory that had been growing among some CTE researchers: Maybe it was not the severe concussions that caused the bulk of the damage. Maybe it was the minor hits, the subconcussive blows that happened on almost every play, that caused CTE.

Nowinski and McKee announced their findings at a press conference in January 2009 in Tampa, Florida, in the middle of the media coverage leading up to Super Bowl XLIII. McHale's family made the announcement, and McKee made a presentation of her findings. "I have never seen this disease in the general population, only in these athletes," she said. "It's a crisis, and anyone who doesn't recognize the severity of the problem is in tremendous denial."[17] The story was covered in the *New York Times* and picked up by major news outlets.

The NFL Is Compared to Big Tobacco

After the Super Bowl, Congress began to take interest in the concussion controversy. A few months later the House Judiciary Committee announced that it would hold hearings to investigate the role of brain damage in professional football. NFL commissioner Roger Goodell, who had succeeded Tagliabue in 2006, appeared in front of the committee and was asked directly if there was a link between football and brain-related injuries. Goodell evaded the issue again and again, stating that he was not a scientist and could not speak to the issue. Finally, Representative Linda Sánchez said, "The N.F.L. sort of has this blanket denial or minimizing of the fact that there may be this link. And it sort of reminds me of the tobacco companies pre-'90s when they kept saying, 'Oh, there's no link between smoking and damage to your health.'"[18] According to the authors of *League of Denial*, the comparison to the tobacco industry in a congressional hearing was a nightmare scenario for the NFL. It gave the public an easy way to understand the concussion controversy: The NFL equals Big Tobacco.

The 2009 congressional hearings marked the beginning of the end of decades of denial by the NFL. Three weeks later Goodell disbanded the MTBI Committee, renaming it the NFL Head, Neck and Spine Committee and inviting many of the field's leading concussion experts to join it. Goodell also instituted a rash of rule changes to protect players' safety. The NFL donated $1 million to the Center for the Study of Traumatic Encephalopathy. And finally, in a telephone interview with the *New York Times*, league spokesperson Greg Aiello admitted that concussions can lead to long-term health problems. It was the first time anyone from the NFL had publicly admitted that concussions had any long-term effects. Dr. Robert Stern, codirector of the Center for the Study of Traumatic Encephalopathy, said, "Mr. Aiello's statement is long overdue. . . . With the NFL taking these recent actions, we are finally at a point to move forward in our research and ultimately solve this important problem."[19]

The Research Continues

The concussion controversy is far from over. More and more former athletes with CTE are dying young, many at their own hands. In 2011 NFL safety Dave Duerson committed suicide, leaving a note asking that his brain be given to the NFL for study. He had shot himself in the chest so his brain would not be damaged. NFL linebacker Junior Seau—who many considered the most dynamic player of his generation—did not leave a suicide note, but in 2012 he also shot himself in the chest, as did American professional baseball player Ryan Freel and NFL player Ray Easterling. Autopsies revealed that all of the athletes had CTE. "Those cases speak to me," McKee told *Frontline*. "I think that means something, that they took their lives that way. I think they wanted people to examine their brains. I think they wanted, on some level, for them to be part of the research."[20]

Facts

- The force of a professional boxer's punch is equivalent to being hit with a 13-pound (6 kg) bowling ball traveling 20 miles per hour (32 kph).

- Sugar Ray Robinson, Joe Frazier, and at least fourteen other well-known boxers have been diagnosed with dementia pugilistica. Muhammad Ali has Parkinson's disease, which is thought to be caused by brain trauma in some cases.

- In 2009 it was discovered that the NFL had secretly commissioned a study that found that the incidence of Alzheimer's and other mental disorders was nineteen times higher in former players than in the general population.

- Of all the brains of former NFL players that have been examined by the Center for the Study of Traumatic Encephalopathy, only one was found not to have evidence of CTE.

- It is now thought that baseball player Lou Gehrig may not have had ALS, a neurodegenerative disease also known as Lou Gehrig's disease. Some doctors now believe Gehrig suffered from concussion-related trauma.

CHAPTER TWO

How Dangerous Are Concussions?

There is a long history of misunderstanding concussions in sports. Many still think a person must lose consciousness to be diagnosed with a concussion. Others believe that concussions are minor injuries that can be shaken off. However, the short-term and long-term damage from concussions can be devastating. Understanding what happens inside the brain during a concussion will help athletes and their coaches recognize and properly treat concussions before the brain is permanently damaged.

What Is a Concussion?

A concussion is a traumatic brain injury caused by an external mechanical force such as a blow to the head. The brain is suspended in cerebrospinal fluid, a clear, colorless bodily fluid that prevents the brain—which is the consistency of soft gelatin—from collapsing under its own weight. It also acts as a cushion, protecting the brain from injury when the body is jolted. However, sometimes the body is jolted with so much force that the fluid cannot prevent the brain from striking the rough interior of the skull. When this occurs, brain function is often affected, and the injury is called a concussion. A person is diagnosed with a concussion if the injury has caused a change in alertness or cognitive function. A mild concussion usually produces a feeling of disorientation and nausea, sometimes referred to as "wooziness" or "seeing stars." A severe concussion results in unconsciousness.

Concussions

As athletes get bigger, stronger, and faster than ever before, concussions—caused by violent collisions—have become a troubling part of many sports.

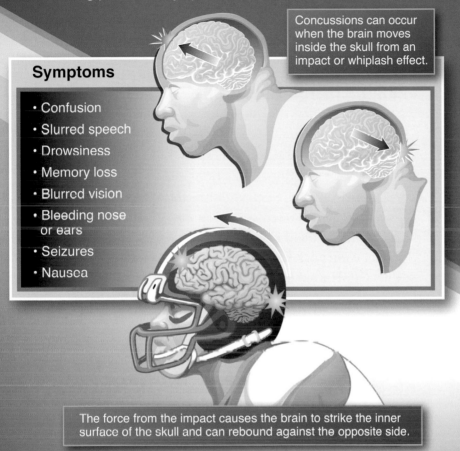

Concussions can occur when the brain moves inside the skull from an impact or whiplash effect.

Symptoms

- Confusion
- Slurred speech
- Drowsiness
- Memory loss
- Blurred vision
- Bleeding nose or ears
- Seizures
- Nausea

The force from the impact causes the brain to strike the inner surface of the skull and can rebound against the opposite side.

Source: National Institutes of Health, "Concussions," 2012. nlm.nih.gov.

It is not necessary to be hit on the head to get a concussion. When the body stops suddenly (such as in a fall) or changes direction rapidly (such as in a car crash), the brain does not; it keeps moving through the cerebrospinal fluid until it hits the inside of the skull. A blow to the head has the same effect—the brain jolts until it strikes one side of the skull, then reverses and strikes the opposite side. While many different kinds of impacts can cause a concussion, those caused by blows to the head, rather than to the body, tend to be much more serious because greater forces on the brain are involved.

In sports, concussions are caused by being struck by an object or by colliding with a piece of equipment, another player, or the ground. Concussions are most common in boxing and in contact team sports like football, rugby, and ice hockey. However, concussions can happen in any sport.

Changes Inside the Brain

When a person sustains a concussion, the brain goes into overdrive, releasing massive amounts of chemicals known as neurotransmitters. Neurotransmitters are the chemicals that the brain uses to send messages from one axon (the strands of fiber that link nerve cells together) to the next. When the brain is injured, it floods the system with neurotransmitters, and communication among the nerve cells becomes overloaded.

In order for the brain to function correctly, it must maintain a chemical balance between potassium ions, which are inside the cells, and calcium ions, which are outside the cells. But once the brain is overloaded, it cannot regulate itself. Calcium ions flood into the cells and potassium ions flood out. The brain tries to clean up the mess of calcium, potassium, and other chemicals, but because it is out of balance, it has trouble making enough energy to do the job. Any strain on the brain—which includes everything from playing sports to watching television—slows down the cleanup process, leaving the brain vulnerable to further damage.

"Kids' heads are almost full size by the age of four, but their musculature obviously isn't, so you get the bobblehead effect on the brain."[21]

— Dr. Ann McKee, codirector of the Center for the Study of Traumatic Encephalopathy.

Kids and Concussions

Children's brains are especially vulnerable to concussions. Scientists are not sure why this is so, but they believe that it is because children do not have the neck muscle strength that adults have. Because they have less musculature, they cannot brace for an im-

Linear and Rotational Forces

Two types of forces cause concussions: linear and rotational. When the skull is hit or jolted in a straight line, such as when a car is rear-ended, this is considered a linear force, which causes a linear acceleration of the brain. The head snaps in a straight line, either front to back or side to side, and the brain does as well, hitting the inside of the skull straight on. When the head or body is hit off center, this is considered a rotational force. This type of impact causes the brain to twist inside the skull and then quickly snap back. Both linear and rotational forces are present to some degree in almost every impact that causes a concussion, but the rotational forces are thought to be much more dangerous. When the brain twists inside the skull, tissue and blood vessels stretch and tear, causing much more overall trauma. Both forces are even more damaging when a person does not brace for the impact. This is why some sports leagues have outlawed blindside, or "defenseless player," hits; a player who is surprised by a hit is much more likely to be injured because his muscles have not tensed to absorb some of the force of the blow.

pact as successfully as an adult can. Another issue is head size. "Kids' heads are almost full size by the age of four, but their musculature obviously isn't, so you get the bobblehead effect on the brain,"[21] explains McKee. This puts younger children at special risk. The larger a child's head is in proportion to his or her body, the greater the risk of concussion.

Children's brains are also still developing. In an adult the axons are coated in a protective sheath called myelin. As neurosurgeon Robert Cantu, codirector of the Center for the Study of Traumatic Encephalopathy, explains, myelin coats axon fibers like a rubber coating coats a copper electrical wire. "The coating insulates, protects, and strengthens that wire. The fiber tracks of adults have a coating of myelin that acts in the same way, protecting the fibers from injury or insult."[22] However, children's brains have less myelin, which makes their brain structures much more vulnerable to damage.

Youth concussions also tend to be more severe than adult concussions, and recovery time is longer. According to neurologist Julian Bailes, medical director for the Pop Warner Youth Football program, because the immature brain is still developing, it is "more susceptible to damage and more likely to suffer repetitive injury."[23] While the average adult will fully recover from a mild concussion within seven to ten days, a young person will often need a full month to be symptom free.

Symptoms of a Concussion

The symptoms for concussion vary from person to person and depend on the seriousness of the injury. They include confusion, dizziness, fatigue, nausea, vomiting, headache, amnesia, and loss of consciousness. Players who sustain minor concussions may not be

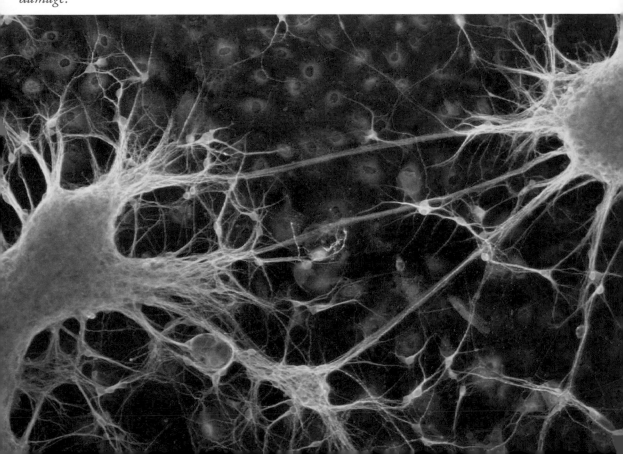

immediately aware of it in the heat of play, and it is the team doctor's or athletic trainer's responsibility to evaluate players who may have been concussed. Doctors ask questions that test whether or not players know what is going on around them. Cantu, who has developed widely used criteria for evaluating concussions, says that he asks questions such as, "What is the play you were injured on? What quarter is it? What is the score?"[24] He also performs a balance test and tests a player's cognitive ability: "I give them six digits and ask them to repeat them, then to repeat them backwards."[25]

Unfortunately, many times the coach or team doctor does not have the training to know how or when to evaluate a player for a concussion. One dramatic example of this was uncovered in a youth ice hockey league in Ontario, Canada. Dr. Paul Echlin attempted to track the number of concussions among the players of two teams during the 2009–2010 season. From the stands, he would note any player that he thought had been concussed and evaluate him in the locker room between periods. At that point, concussions were reported to occur at a rate of 3.1 concussions per 1,000 man-games (12 players in one game equals 12 man-games). However, Echlin counted 21.5 concussions per 1,000 man-games—seven times the number of concussions that were typically reported. In his study, Echlin reported that concussed players claimed they were sometimes pressured by their coaches or their parents to return to play even when medical professionals had advised them to take time off. In fact, one father told Echlin's group members that they should leave because his son "needs to play on instincts and can't be worried about getting a concussion every time he goes into a corner."[26] Echlin concluded that the pressure to win was blinding the adults to the dangers of concussions and that "the athlete has to be educated about the long-term seriousness of concussion and encouraged to self-report."[27]

"[My son] needs to play on instincts and can't be worried about getting a concussion every time he goes into a corner."[26]

— The father of a player in a youth ice hockey league.

Recovering from a Concussion

There is no cure for a concussion except for mental and physical rest. The brain must devote all of its resources to repairing itself.

To help sports leagues determine when it is safe for a player to return to the sport, Cantu and other experts have developed Return to Play guidelines. For instance, in Cantu's guidelines, a player who suffers one mild concussion (defined as a concussion in which there is no loss of consciousness and all concussion symptoms disappear within thirty minutes) may return to play in one week. A second concussion requires a longer rest period and sometimes requires leaving the sport for the season, and a third concussion, according to Cantu, always requires quitting for the season. A rest period does not just mean physical rest; the player must eliminate any intellectually stimulating activity. "This includes any activity that involves staring at a screen or a page,"[28] says Cantu, including engaging in any Internet or texting activities, watching TV and movies, and excessive reading.

The reason that each concussion demands an increasingly longer rest period is that concussion damage seems to be cumulative. The biggest risk factor for getting a concussion is having had a concussion in the past. A player who returns to play too soon after a concussion can acquire another one from a minor impact—or even from being jostled by another player. Scientists are not sure why, but studies show that the first concussion somehow primes the brain to be vulnerable to the second.

"She'd woken up to [see] me standing on the bed, sweating profusely, trying to climb the wall. Eventually I jumped headfirst into the wall and went through the nightstand."[29]

— Former professional wrestler Chris Nowinski.

Post-Concussion Syndrome

Some players—especially those who have sustained multiple concussions—acquire post-concussion syndrome, a debilitating condition that affects every aspect of daily life. Symptoms include severe headaches; sleep problems; mood problems such as depression, irritability, and anxiety; and problems with memory, concentration, and thinking. When Chris Nowinski was wrestling in the WWF, a series of concussions left him with post-concussion syndrome and forced him to leave the sport. As he tells *Frontline*, on the night he decided to quit, "I woke up on the floor of the hotel room surrounded by a broken nightstand and lamp, and my girlfriend screaming in the corner because she told me she'd woken up to me standing on the bed, sweating profusely, trying to climb the wall. Eventually I jumped headfirst into the wall and went through the nightstand."[29] Nowinski suffered a variety of cognitive and psychological difficulties. He also had severe headaches for five years and sleep disturbances for three.

Second-Impact Syndrome

Another devastating result of multiple concussions is second-impact syndrome (SIS). SIS can occur when a person—almost always a teenager—suffers a second concussion before having fully recovered from the first. In SIS the brain undergoes massive cerebral edema after the second concussion, swelling rapidly inside the skull. The swelling crushes the brain's blood vessels inside the skull, which is usually fatal. The condition is rare—only about thirty cases have been reported in the medical literature. One victim of SIS was seventeen-year-old Nathan Stiles, a straight-A student and the homecoming king of his Kansas high school. Stiles died of SIS after receiving a trivial hit in a football game. He had suffered a concussion about a month before, but after a clean CAT scan and a three-week rest period, he had been cleared to play by his family physician. Right before halftime of his final game of his senior year, Stiles collapsed on the sidelines and began having a seizure. He was airlifted to the hospital, and although doctors were able to stop the bleeding inside his brain, he had suffered too much trauma and was taken off life support later that night.

Chronic Traumatic Encephalopathy

Stiles was also the youngest person whose brain had signs of CTE, the neurodegenerative disease that destroys brain cells and causes dementia in later life. The main characteristic of the disease is a proliferation of the protein tau in the brain tissue. Tau is a protein found inside nerve cell axons. Scientists believe that when a concussion damages the axons, tau is released. If the brain is not given time to heal and clean itself, the tau becomes poisonous and gradually spreads through the brain, destroying brain cells. Tau appears on prepared slides as brown tangles, which clog the brain tissue. Because tau tangles are also a feature of Alzheimer's disease,

Return-to-Play Guidelines

While many return-to-play guidelines exist, those developed by Dr. Robert Cantu are used most frequently by team doctors. Many professional and collegiate leagues base their concussion policies on Cantu's guidelines.

	First Concussion	Second Concussion	Third Concussion
No loss of consciousness **or** signs/symptoms clear in 30 minutes	May return to play after 1 week if asymptomatic at rest and during progressive exertion protocol.	May return to play in 2 weeks if asymptomatic for 1 week at rest and during progressive exertion protocol.	Terminate season; may return to play next season if asymptomatic at rest and during progressive exertion protocol.
Loss of consciousness for less than 1 minute **or** more than 30 minutes posttraumatic amnesia **or** signs/symptoms last less than 1 week	May return to play if asymptomatic for 1 week and during progressive exertion protocol.	Out for a minimum of 1 month; may return to play if asymptomatic for 1 week at rest and during progressive exertion protocol; consider terminating season.	Terminate season; may return to play next season if asymptomatic at rest and during progressive exertion protocol.
Loss of consciousness for 1 minute or longer **or** more than 24 hours of posttraumatic amnesia **or** signs/symptoms last more than 7 days	Out for a minimum of 1 month; may return to play AFTER 4 weeks if asymptomatic for 1 week at rest and during progressive exertion protocol.	Terminate season; may return to play next season if asymptomatic at rest and during progressive exertion protocol.	

Source: Sports Legacy Institute, Cantu's Return-to-Play Guidelines, www.sportslegacy.org/policy/return-to-play.

scientists know that it is responsible for the dementia that accompanies CTE.

McKee and Cantu recently conducted a study of the brain samples of eighty-five people, including Stiles, who had experienced concussions and other mild traumatic brain injury during their lives—mostly from athletics. Sixty-eight of them had CTE. Some of them, including twenty-one-year-old Owen Thomas, had never had a concussion, only the subconcussive blows associated with contact sports. As McKee explains, "The trauma usually is experienced early in life, in the teens and twenties, and people develop symptoms years later, often after they retire from the sports. . . . As long as the person lives the symptoms get worse. It's usually a long, steady decline."[30] Symptoms of CTE include aggression, impulsivity, problems with thinking and concentration, memory loss, and depression. Depression can lead to suicide—as was the case with Thomas. McKee and the research team concluded, "This study clearly shows that . . . there may be severe and devastating long-term consequences of repetitive brain trauma that has traditionally been considered only mild."[31]

Cause of CTE in Dispute

Despite work by McKee and Cantu, some researchers still do not think it has been established that concussions cause CTE. Among them are neuropsychologists Stella Karantzoulis and Christopher Randolph, who recently published a study that argued that the evidence linking concussion and CTE is limited. They argue that suicide, which is considered a key feature of CTE, is actually less common among retired NFL players than it is in the general population. They also argue that abnormal tau deposits may not be a reliable way to diagnose CTE, citing case studies that indicate that between 20 and 50 percent of people who had abnormal tau deposits in their brains did not have any symptoms of CTE. They write, "There currently are no carefully controlled data, however, to indicate a definitive association between sport-related concussion and increased risk for late-life cognitive and neuropsychiatric impairment of any form."[32] These scientists are not alone. In 2012 at the Fourth International Conference on Concussion in Sport, medical experts released a consensus statement that said: "A cause and effect relationship has not as yet been demonstrated between CTE and concussions or exposure to contact sports."[33]

McKee disagrees. "We've never seen this disease in a person who didn't have substantial dramatic exposure [to brain injury]," she said to an audience at Samford University in Alabama. "You'll notice that none of my critics are ever neuropathologists because neuropathologists know what you find in people's brains even if

Concussing a Mouse

A mistake by an eighteen-year-old intern allowed scientists to look at a living brain right after a concussion. Theo Roth, who was interning at the National Institutes of Health, was given the task of shaving down the skulls of unconscious mice so that the bone would be nearly transparent under a lighted microscope. However, Roth kept accidently giving the mice concussions. This mistake allowed the scientists to see that after a concussion, there is a quick buildup of free radicals that leak through the membrane that encases the brain. Free radicals are part of the inflammatory response, but when they come in contact with brain tissue, they destroy it.

The scientists then tried to prevent the damage to the brain with antioxidants, which fight free radicals. Roth put a drop of the antioxidant gluthathione on the porous bone of a mouse's skull. By the next morning, the process had worked—there was no detectable injury. Subsequent tests showed that, on average, antioxidants prevent 70 percent of the damage to the brain. The study was published in the January 2014 edition of the journal *Nature*. Because of the young intern's mistake, doctors may soon be able to treat concussions with an antioxidant patch placed on the skull right after the injury.

they live to be 100. This is very abnormal. The fact that we've even seen it with people who are head bangers speaks to the fact this is a traumatic disease."[34] (McKee was referring to an autistic person with a history of banging her head who was included in the study.) McKee, Cantu, and Nowinski do agree that much more research needs to be done on CTE so that the risks can be understood. "I think we're going to find that football poses a risk to our children that we're not comfortable with," Nowinski told *Frontline*. "And it all depends on how fast and how far we move to change it before this day of reckoning comes."[35]

One problem with current research is that most of the autopsies that test for CTE are done on athletes who suffered from CTE symptoms while they were alive. "It's a very skewed sample of brains that we look at," notes Cantu. "So the fact that we have found such a high incidence of CTE is partially explained by the fact that these were very symptomatic people."[36] Controlled studies are needed to fully understand the relationship between sports concussions, tau, and CTE. One of the questions researchers are asking is why tau shows up in the brain of someone as young as seventeen-year-old Nathan Stiles, yet many older ex-athletes with a history of concussion have no symptoms of the disease. "Clearly, there's genetic variability here," says Cantu. "We're trying to identify those genetic factors, so that if a kid tests positive for the markers, his parents can hold him out of contact sports."[37] The Center for the Study of Traumatic Encephalopathy is currently conducting a study that may do just that. The DETECT Study seeks to develop ways of detecting CTE during life. It will include 150 former NFL players, as well as a control group of 50 athletes who played noncontact sports. The study was expected to be completed in 2015.

Recent Breakthroughs

Research on the damaging effects of concussions has been progressing rapidly in the past few years. In 2013 a study of three different college football teams found that after each practice, a brain protein called S100B showed up in the players' blood. "The only way S100B can find its way into the blood is if the gate between the brain and the blood is open,"[38] explained study coauthor Dr. Jeffrey Bazarian. The blood-brain barrier is a membrane that keeps dangerous chemicals from invading the brain. "We think that just playing football, even without getting a concussion, can open the blood-brain barrier,"[39] Bazarian said. In the study the more hits to the head a player sustained, the higher the levels of S100B. The researchers were concerned that if S100B could break through the blood-brain barrier, the brain would be vulnerable to attack (and damage) by antibodies that recognize S100B as a foreign invader.

Bazarian and his colleagues believe that a blood test for S100B performed on the field could alert players to these dangerous leaks in their blood-brain barrier.

Another breakthrough was made by Julian Bailes and Bennet Omalu at the Brain Injury Research Institute. In 2013 they were able to detect tau protein in the living brains of eight former NFL players who had been complaining of symptoms of CTE. The researchers were testing a radioactive marker that clings to tau protein deposits inside the brain, allowing the deposits to show up on brain scans. "Identifying CTE in a living person is the holy grail for this disease and for us to be able to make advances in treatment,"[40] said Bailes. However, the researchers warn that the study sample is very small and there is still a lot to learn.

While research into sports, concussions, tau, and CTE is progressing, all involved agree that it must advance as quickly as possible. "We need to do something now, this minute," says McKee, who spends as much time as she can educating the public about the brain damage she sees in her lab. "Too many kids are at risk."[41]

Facts

- A 2010 study published in the *American Journal of Sports Medicine* found that less than 10 percent of concussions involve a loss of consciousness.

- Scientists estimate that the impact an NFL lineman undergoes during a typical play is equivalent to driving a car 35 miles per hour (56 kph) into a brick wall.

- The Sports Legacy Institute estimates that NFL linemen undergo about one thousand to thirteen hundred subconcussive blows to the head per season, and that some male ice hockey players receive nearly one thousand blows to the head per season.

- An informal survey of 261 pro baseball catchers performed by Los Angeles Dodgers trainer Stan Conte in 2006 found that 20–25 percent of catchers had experienced concussion symptoms from being hit with foul balls.

- NASCAR did not add baseline neurological testing for concussions until the 2014 season.

- According to the 2012 Sports Concussion Consensus Conference, amateur horse racing has the highest incidence of concussion, at 95.2 concussions per one thousand player hours.

- The Sports Concussion Institute reports that 47 percent of athletes do not report feeling any symptoms immediately after a concussive blow.

CHAPTER THREE

Are Adult Leagues Doing Enough to Protect Players?

I n all sports, protecting players from concussions can occur in two areas. First, the incidence of concussion can be reduced through changes to equipment, rules of play, and behavior on the field. Second, the damage done by a concussion can be reduced by improving treatment protocols. The NFL has led the way in reducing concussion risk, and many of its methods have been adopted by other adult sports leagues. However, there are still critics on both sides: Some think that sports leagues have not done enough to keep players safe, while others think that efforts to make sports safer diminish their appeal.

Football Rule Changes Have Made Play Safer

Over the past decade, the NFL has made a slew of rule changes to help prevent hits to the head and neck. Various "defenseless player" rules make it illegal to hit players in the head and neck when they are not braced for it, such as when a receiver is in the process of catching the ball. Other rules prevent players from charging each other headfirst or using their helmets as weapons during tackles. The NFL has also instituted a hit count during practice, which limits the number of head and body hits a player can sustain. It has also reduced the amount of time a team can spend on tackling drills to limit exposure to concussion risk. The National Collegiate Athletic Association (NCAA) has adopted many of these rules, and individual schools often develop policies in their football programs that are even more conservative than NCAA standards.

One of the NFL's most significant rule changes was made to the kickoff. Kickoff returns—which occur at the start of each half of play—are the most injury-fraught plays in professional football. The players, who are sprinting toward each other from opposite ends of the field, collide with far more force than they do on other plays. In 2011 Roger Goodell moved the kickoff spot forward 5 yards (4.6 m), from the 30- to the 35-yard line, and moved the players' starting positions forward as well. These two changes had a profound effect, reducing concussions on kickoff plays by 40 percent. The NCAA adopted NFL kickoff rules in 2012 and also saw its total incidence of concussion go down dramatically. The change was so successful that Goodell has said he is considering eliminating the kickoff altogether.

Criticism of Rule Changes

The change in kickoff rules has gotten a great deal of criticism from football fans, who claim that it reduces the excitement of the kickoff return play. In addition, many kickoff plays are now ended prematurely because the kicker is more likely to kick the ball into the end zone, allowing the receiving team to start on its 20-yard line without running the ball. However, in some circumstances the new rule is having the opposite effect, prompting kickoff returners to make risky runs rather than end the play. "Guys who are returners, they get paid to be returners. That's how they're making their money and it's how they're supporting their family," explains Buffalo Bills kicker Dan Carpenter. "They're willing to take more risks on bringing the ball out."[42]

The kickoff is not the only rule change that has drawn criticism. Many fans and players are also frustrated that hits that were once legal are now illegal, drawing penalties and fines of $75,000 and up. Many of these changes were made to protect the quarterback—a practice that has drawn especially intense criticism. "The degree to which the NFL has gone to make the game easier on quarterbacks borders on sickening,"[43] commentator Gus Turner writes, referring to a rule that made it illegal to tackle a quarterback below the knee. Critics like Turner claim that defensive players are being restricted in unrealistic ways, forcing them to change tactics in the middle of a play to avoid making illegal hits. They also claim that these rule changes weaken the physicality of the sport in unacceptable ways. "They change the rules a lot," said New York Giants running back David Wilson. "I think there is only so much you can modify the game until it turns into a different sport."[44]

Diagnosis and Return to Play

Nearly every major league sport in the United States has an established policy for dealing with concussions. All of these policies include conducting yearly baseline testing to establish a player's normal brain function. Most use the Immediate Post-Concussion Assessment and Cognitive Testing (ImPACT) program for baseline and post-concussion testing, a computer-based cognitive test that can be administered on the sidelines. However, although the program is extremely useful for capturing, tracking, and evaluating cognitive performance before and after a concussion, its results can be misleading if they are not evaluated by a physician knowledgeable about concussions. Results can also be manipulated by the players. In fact, some NFL players have recently admitted that they deliberately try to do poorly on their baseline tests so they will be less likely to be benched for a concussion.

The NFL's concussion policy was developed by its Head, Neck and Spine Committee and is posted on the NFL's website. Players are monitored on the field by an athletic trainer, who watches television replays for possible concussions. Players are then assessed by the team doctor and a neuro-trauma expert unaffiliated with the NFL. If the player is diagnosed with a possible concussion, he must leave the field for the remainder of the game. The NFL does not have a prescribed period of recovery; rather, it monitors the player throughout the recuperation period. "The thing that I think is im-

"The degree to which the NFL has gone to make the game easier on quarterbacks borders on sickening."[43]

— Commentator Gus Turner.

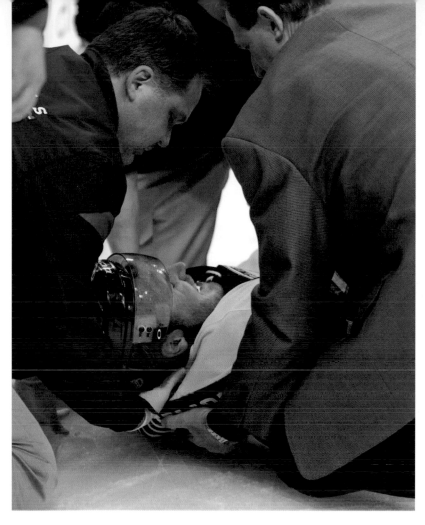

NHL player James Wisniewski is attended to by medical staff after an injury. Wisniewski is one of several professional athletes who have admitted concealing concussion symptoms to avoid being benched or replaced.

portant here is you don't manage concussions by a calendar," said Dr. Stan Herring, a member of the Head, Neck, and Spine Committee. "Some guys may come back in a week. Some guys may come back in six weeks. These steps don't have an expiration date on them. The player's history of injury and other issues come into play."[45]

Problems with Measuring Success

Although Goodell has been praised for taking a strong stance against concussions, it is difficult to tell if their incidence is being reduced—in part because it is not clear how many concussions are actually occurring. For instance, from 2010 to 2013 the Oakland Raiders reported thirty-two player concussions, whereas the Houston Texans reported only three. According to former defensive back Jeff Nixon at the *Nixon Report*, this is not because the Texans have fewer concussions; it is because the Raiders have been more proactive about reporting them. Nixon also points out that the language of injury reports is inconsistent. A player can be reported as having a head injury when he actually has a concussion. Nixon says this is because some teams have a tendency "to flout the protocol around benching players with brain injuries, in part by calling their injuries something that isn't a 'concussion.'"[46] He suggests that both terminology and injury response should be standardized for player safety.

Concussions Persist in Ice Hockey

In 2011 the National Hockey League (NHL) followed the NFL's lead by banning all hits to the head. To measure whether the change reduced the incidence of concussions, neurosurgeon Michael Cusimano conducted a study of three seasons of NHL play—one before and two after the rule change. Surprisingly, the incidence of concussions went up each year: There were forty-four concussions before the rule change and sixty-five and eighty-five in the two years after the rule change. More than 64 percent of concussions were due to legal body checking. This practice may have even more risk of concussion than blows to the head because of the whiplash effect, which often causes the brain to twist inside the skull, and because players often hit their heads on the boards that surround the rink. Cusimano, a lifelong hockey fan, would like to see body checking banned entirely. "I don't think there's really a big advantage of checking in professional hockey, if you look at things like the all-star game, where body-checking is rare but play is still exciting,"[47] he said.

Players Hide Injuries

Sometimes it is the players themselves who put themselves in harm's way by hiding their concussions. Despite the NFL's commitment to safety, players can still find themselves out of a job because of an injury. San Francisco 49ers quarterback Alex Smith found this out when he self-reported a concussion and was permanently replaced—even though he was having the best season of his career. Incidents like this only encourage players to hide concussions, as New York Jets quarterback Greg McElroy did in 2012. After being sacked eleven times in a 2012 game against the San Diego Chargers, he hid his concussion symptoms from trainers for four days because he did not want to be benched.

A similar incident occurred in 2014 in the NHL. After being body checked so violently that he had to be helped off the ice, James Wisniewski of the Columbus Blue Jackets returned to play in the next period. Wisniewski—who had suffered a significant brain injury the season before—later admitted, "I said my back hurt so I didn't have to do the 20-minute (concussion) protocol and go through that whole concussion process. I didn't feel like going in and talking to the doctors for 20 minutes. A lot of guys were playing through [injuries]. . . . That's playoff hockey. It's survival of the fittest."[48] Neither the NFL nor the NHL have any effective solutions to this problem. Both sports make player substitutions that are in a team's best interest, and players who are injured have no guarantee that they will not be replaced.

"I said my back hurt so I didn't have to do the 20-minute (concussion) protocol and go through that whole concussion process."[48]

— NHL player James Wisniewski.

Helmets Are Mostly Ineffective

The NFL has been attempting to prevent concussions through improved helmet design for decades. Its latest effort is a $10 million incentive program called the Head Health Challenge, which it launched in 2013 in partnership with General Electric. Although one of the program's missions was to find better shock-absorbent material for helmets, it has not yet awarded funds to any researchers working on that problem. This may be because studies have consistently shown that, although helmets are excellent at reducing the impact of lateral forces—such as from a ball or a stick—they do not reduce the rotational forces that twist the brain and cause the most serious concussions in contact sports. In a 2014 study, researchers from Florida State University analyzed ten popular football helmet designs and found that, on average, they were only 20 percent more effective at preventing concussion than wearing no helmet at all. Study author Dr. Frank Condi said:

Biomechanics researchers have long understood that rotational forces, not linear forces, are responsible for serious brain damage including concussion, brain injury complications and brain bleeds. Yet generations of football and other sports participants have been under the assumption that their brains are protected by their investment in headwear protection.[49]

Because helmets can make players feel more protected than they are, some are debating whether helmets should be eliminated from football altogether. Ainissa Ramirez, coauthor of *Newton's Football*, argues that removing helmets would automatically make the game safer because players would be more protective of their heads. She explains that football players only began leading with their heads after the introduction of the face mask in 1953, which protected their face from injury. In fact, both former Chicago Bears coach Mike Ditka and the late Penn State Nittany Lions coach Joe Paterno have argued that simply removing the face mask from the helmet would reduce head injury. As Paterno explained, without the face mask "you would get back to shoulder blocking and shoulder tackling and you wouldn't have all these heroes out there."[50] However, critics argue that although the helmet may not be useful at preventing concussions, it is excellent at protecting the brain from severe trauma. Robert Cantu points out that between 1961 and 1970—before helmet safety standards were put in place—there were 244 fatalities in football, almost all of them due to head and neck injuries. In 1968 alone there were thirty-eight deaths—twenty-six in high school football. "Removing helmets from football players would reduce the incidence of concussion but would replace it with an epidemic of skull fractures and subdural hematoma deaths,"[51] Cantu asserts.

> "Generations of football and other sports participants have been under the assumption that their brains are protected by their investment in headwear protection."[49]
>
> — Dr. Frank Condi.

Helmet Sensors Aid Researchers

One helmet innovation funded by sports leagues that has proved to be extremely useful is helmet sensors. Dr. Kevin Guskiewicz,

Concussion Controversy During Soccer's World Cup

During a 2014 World Cup game, Uruguay midfielder Alvaro Pereira was briefly knocked unconscious. The team doctor performed a quick examination and then called for a player substitution. But when Pereira insisted he was able to play, the doctor returned him to the game. Concussion advocate Taylor Twellman called the incident "barbaric." "When a player is concussed he doesn't know what has happened," he said. "[It's] very dangerous to rely on what a player wants." Twellman claims that international soccer lags far behind other sports when it comes to concussion management.

One problem is with the rules of play. According to international soccer rules, all player substitutions are permanent. Doctors have only a minute or two to test for concussion before they must decide whether to bench a player for the rest of the game. When players insist they are fine—as Pereira did—doctors sometimes take their word for it. According FIFPro, the international soccer players' union, "Teams and players should not be disadvantaged for upholding player health and safety, or encouraged to act in a way that compromises it." FIFPro has called for rule changes that make international concussion protocols mandatory and allow for temporary medical substitutions.

Quoted in Kieran Murray, "Uruguay's Knocked-Out Pereira Admits 'Madness' of Playing On," Reuters, June 19, 2014. www.reuters.com.

Quoted in the Associated Press, "At World Cup, Calls for Better Management of Concussions and Possible Rule Changes," Fox News, June 23, 2014. www.foxnews.com.

who has been researching helmet performance and concussions since his days as an athletic trainer with the Pittsburgh Steelers, uses the Head Impact Telemetry (HIT) system to study football impacts. The HIT system places specialized sensors inside the football helmet to measure the frequency and intensity of linear and rotational forces. The system is at use in several universities, including Virginia Tech, Brown, and Dartmouth, but at $50,000 to $60,000 per team, it is cost-prohibitive for most colleges. Although the NFL supports the use of the HIT system in practices and games, the NFL Players Association has rejected its use for years because of concerns that HIT data might be used to evaluate performance.

The HIT system has revealed new information about concussions. Before Guskiewicz's research, doctors thought that concussions usually happened at forces above 85 g. (G-force is a measurement of acceleration felt as weight. One g is equivalent to the pull of gravity of a person standing on the earth.) However, when Guskiewicz tracked the North Carolina State University football team for five seasons using the HIT system, he found that six out of the thirteen concussions measured occurred at or below 85 g. "People see massive hits and think, 'That's the one,' and ignore the more trivial blows,"[52] Guskiewicz explained.

Guskiewicz also found that most concussions are caused by impacts to the crown of the head, rather than from side impacts, as was previously thought. This knowledge allowed him to educate the North Carolina team on how to hit safely. He videotaped players and showed them how different techniques would allow them to hit harder without sustaining concussions. For instance, Melik Brown had sustained two concussions on typical blocking moves because he lowered his head before impact. After seeing the video and being instructed on form, Brown was able to hit much harder with no harm to himself. "The video shows him rotating his head out of the way just before impact," Guskiewicz explains. "His shoulder pads absorbed most of the blow. This is just one case, but it shows that there's a lot more to concussions than just force of impact."[53]

Heading the Ball in Soccer

Soccer has also come under scrutiny for its concussion risk. While the risk of concussions in soccer has not been well studied, a sur-

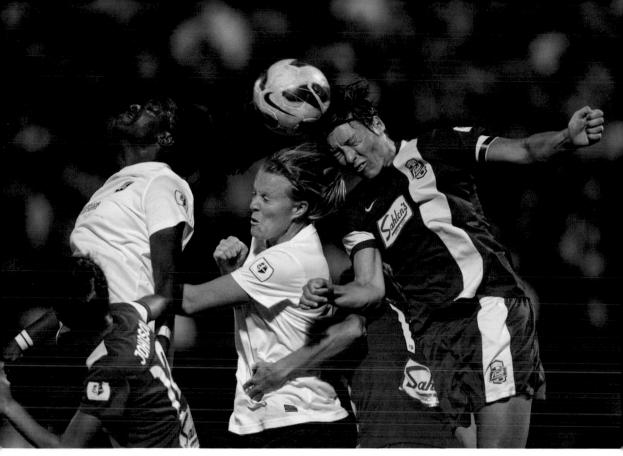

vey at McGill University in Quebec, Canada, found that more than 60 percent of college soccer players reported symptoms of concussions during the regular season. Concussions are usually caused by collisions between players, which often happens when two or more players try to head the ball at the same time. However, research is indicating that heading the ball in itself may carry risk. A recent study of thirty-seven amateur adult soccer players found that the players who headed the ball 885 to 1,550 times a year had nerve cell damage in their brains, and those who headed the ball more than 1,800 times had lower memory scores. This indicates that it is the repetitive subconcussive blows caused by heading the ball, rather than concussion damage, that causes brain changes in soccer players.

Like the NFL and the NHL, US professional soccer leagues conduct baseline brain function testing at the beginning of each season and have established Return to Play policies and proce-

Research has suggested that the soccer tactic of heading the ball causes nerve cell damage in the brains of players who perform it frequently.

dures when treating concussions. However, they have done little to prevent concussion risk in the sport. Since heading the ball is an integral part of play, few are calling for its elimination at the adult level. Soccer advocates have noted that, so far, research studies are too small to make any conclusion about the link between heading the ball and brain damage.

Even so, several head guards have entered the market that are designed to reduce the risk of head injury from collision. Most of these guards are constructed like padded headbands, leaving the top of the head bare. However, one research study found that the guards did not provide any substantial protection against concussions, and there are no signs that college or adult leagues will be requiring them for play.

US Soccer, the governing body for soccer in the United States, has recently announced that it will establish a chief medical officer position in order to better interface with experts in concussion management and prevention in the medical community. US Soccer and Major League Soccer have also announced that they will jointly organize a medical summit to coordinate their efforts to prevent and manage concussions. They also plan to launch a campaign to educate the public about concussion risk and prevention.

Combat Sports and Concussions

Boxing is one of the only major adult sports that does not have an established Return to Play concussion policy—in part because the object of combat sports such as boxing and mixed martial arts is to cause brain and body trauma. A knockout, after all, is the result of a severe concussion with loss of consciousness. Removing deliberate concussive blows from boxing would essentially eliminate boxing as a sport.

Because brain trauma is inherently unsafe, medical groups such as the American Medical Association have been calling for the elimination of boxing and other combat sports since 1982. Even former Naval Academy boxer Senator John McCain called for the ban of mixed martial arts in 1998, calling it the equivalent of "human cock fighting."[54] McCain has since recanted this statement, in part because he was impressed with the way boxing and mixed martial arts are supporting the Professional Fighters Brain Health Study at the Cleveland Clinic Lou Ruvo Center for Brain Health. The study is attempting to develop methods of detecting early brain injury, as well as to understand why some fighters develop chronic neurological disorders and some do not.

Boxing has made various changes over the years to protect fighters from injury, but it is now thought that some of those

Amateur Boxing Bans Headgear

On June 1, 2013, the International Amateur Boxing Association banned the use of headgear in men's amateur boxing competitions. "There's no evidence protective gear shows a reduction in incidence of concussion," said Charles Butler of the association. "In 1982, when the American Medical Association moved to ban boxing, everybody panicked and put headgear on the boxers, but nobody ever looked to see what the headgear did."

In a study published in the *British Journal of Sports Medicine* that examined fifteen thousand boxers, those who wore headgear had a concussion rate of 0.38 percent, whereas those who did not had a rate of 0.17 percent. It turned out that headgear obscures vision, which makes it harder to avoid hits to the side of the head. Researchers also speculate that opponents do not strike as forcefully when headgear is not used. The study concluded that there was "no good evidence that mouthguards and helmets ward off concussion." Headgear will still be worn by youth and female boxers, in part because it is thought that neither group punches with enough force to cause concussions.

Quoted in Kirk Jenness, "Cautionary Tale for MMA: Olympic Boxing Drops Headgear, Adds 10 Pt Must Scoring," *Mixed Martial Arts News*, March 24, 2013. www.mixedmartialarts.com.

changes actually increase the incidence of concussion. For instance, adding padded gloves to protect the hands allows a boxer to punch for a much longer period of time, increasing the blows to the head in any given match. The padding also dramatically increases the concussive power of a punch. And while boxing referees do an excellent job of monitoring a boxer's condition and protecting him or her from serious injury, they can inadvertently increase the number of concussive and subconcussive blows boxers receive. For instance, in most bouts referees have the ability to halt the match at any time for about eight seconds so that a boxer can recover and the referee can evaluate his or her condition. However, this protective count—also called a standing 8 count—often results in bouts that last longer, increasing the chance of concussion and the number of subconcussive blows received by each fighter.

More to Be Done

In the past several years, the NFL has taken the lead in concussion prevention and management by supporting research and being proactive in preventing injury. Most other adult leagues have followed its example and adapted its policies to fit their sport, with varying degrees of success. However, many critics say that much more needs to be done. Some assert that concussions are simply too dangerous to justify the existence of contact sports like football and ice hockey. As commentator Matt Taibbi writes, "As long as it's legal . . . for world-class athletes to run into each other at full speed, concussions are going to be unacceptably common."[55]

Facts

- According to the NCAA Injury Surveillance System, men's soccer players are the fifth-most-likely athletes in all of sports to sustain in-game concussions.

- In 2012 semipro soccer player Patrick Grange died of ALS at age twenty-nine. He was diagnosed in autopsy with CTE. Grange was a prolific header.

- Many semipro football leagues do not require their players to meet any health or equipment standards.

- In 2013 twenty-three Major League Baseball players were put on the league's seven-day concussion disabled list.

- In 2013 the NFL reported that 228 concussions were diagnosed during the season, down from 261 concussions the previous season.

- In the 2013–2014 season, only ten National Basketball Association players were diagnosed with concussions.

- In 2014 the White House announced that the NCAA and the Department of Defense will conduct a study of up to thirty-seven thousand college athletes, the most comprehensive concussion study to date.

CHAPTER FOUR

Are Schools and Youth Leagues Doing Enough to Protect Kids?

L ike many towns in Texas, Marshall loves football. Its well-regarded high school football team, the Marshall Mavericks, has produced several NFL players, and each time it has competed for the state championship, scores of townspeople traveled with the team all the way to Houston and Dallas. But Marshall is now notable for another reason. In February 2014 the school board voted to change its seventh-grade, entry-level tackle football program to flag football—a variation of the game in which players pull Velcro flags off the opposing team instead of tackling them. The measure lets players spend a year developing skills before they started tackling. There was surprisingly little objection from board members or the public. This change in thinking indicates a larger trend in America—more and more parents are questioning the safety of contact sports and wondering if they are worth the risk of concussion. As Marshall resident Matt Moore explains, "I love the game, but I understand it's completely

> "I love the game, but I understand it's completely dangerous and I don't want [my son] to get a life-altering injury."[56]
>
> — Marshall, Texas, resident Matt Moore.

dangerous and I don't want [my son] to get a life-altering injury."[56]

What happened in Marshall is happening all across the country. The effect of sports concussions on America's youth is now a front-and-center topic for parents. Many are taking their children out of sports altogether. Overall enrollment in youth sports has declined, and participation in youth football has dropped nearly 10 percent since 2010. Others are demanding changes in their children's sports programs, and leagues and school districts are trying to find ways to increase safety without changing the sports themselves. This is not always possible, however—as more information about the effect of concussions on young brains comes to light, towns like Marshall are eliminating contact sports for their youngest players. Critics complain that soon, all young athletes will be playing watered-down versions of adult sports and will miss out on college scholarships and future careers in professional leagues.

The White House Gets Involved

To facilitate research and education about youth sports concussions, in May 2014 the White House held its first-ever Healthy Kids and Safe Sports Concussion Summit. The event brought together sports leagues, coaches, parents, medical professionals, and young athletes to raise awareness of concussions and youth sports. One of those athletes was eighteen-year-old Victoria Bellucci, who introduced President Barack Obama. Bellucci suffered five concussions during her high school soccer career, and she had just turned down a soccer scholarship to Towson University because of her struggle with post-concussion syndrome. "It changes the way you think and feel," she told the *Washington Post*. "I was just like really sad, really kind of desperate type of feeling. I couldn't do anything because of my head, so I would just be in my room with the shades drawn. I was like, 'I don't want to live like this anymore.'"[57]

The White House summit highlighted the seriousness of concussions in youth sports. For young people ages fifteen to twenty-four, sports are the second-leading cause of traumatic brain injury—behind only motor vehicle crashes. Each year, al-

"I couldn't do anything because of my head, so I would just be in my room with the shades drawn. I was like,' I don't want to live like this anymore.'"[57]

— Eighteen-year-old former soccer player Victoria Bellucci.

most 250,000 young people visit an emergency room with traumatic brain injuries caused by sports or recreational activities. Experts estimate that at least another 250,000 sustain concussions that are treated by their family doctors—or that are simply not treated at all. And in youth football, at least fifty players have either died or sustained serious brain injuries since 1997—many of them victims of second-impact syndrome.

As Obama pointed out in his opening remarks at the summit, there are too many gaps in scientists' understanding of how concussions affect young people. "Communities are wondering how young . . . to start tackle football," he said. "Parents are wondering whether their kids are learning the right techniques, or wearing the best safety equipment, or whether they should have their kids participate in any full-contact sports at all."[58] These questions are fundamental to the concussion debate. While society has a responsibility to provide for the safety of all athletes, it has a special responsibility to young people, whose futures may be changed forever by sports concussions.

Girls and Concussions

For reasons scientists do not completely understand, girls are especially prone to concussions. Their injuries tend to be more severe than boys' and their recovery time longer. For instance, in high school lacrosse, the concussion rate for girls is twice as high as the rate for boys, even though girls' lacrosse does not allow deliberate contact, or body checking, and boys' lacrosse does. In high school basketball the risk to girls is three times as high as the risk to boys. Competitive cheerleading is perhaps the most dangerous of all extracurricular activities for girls, especially in recent years as aerial maneuvers have become more and more popular. In 2011 thirty-seven thousand cheerleaders were taken to the emergency room after being injured during competition or practice. Many of these injuries were to the skull, caused by being dropped or kicked during an aerial maneuver. Only high school football players suffer more catastrophic injuries. And the flyer on a cheerleading team—the person who is thrown in the air or dismounts from 20 feet (6 m) or more above the ground—is ten times more likely to get a concussion than a football player.

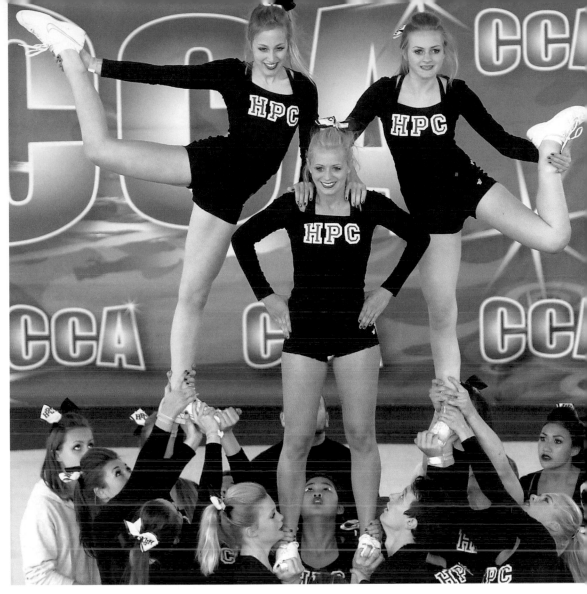

High school cheerleaders perform an aerial maneuver. Although such maneuvers are popular, they can result in a catastrophic injury if a cheerleader is dropped or kicked during one.

Youth Soccer Is Not a Risk-Free Sport

The sport with the highest risk of concussion for girls is soccer. As Lauren Long, former soccer player and cofounder of Concussion Connection, explains it, "I play soccer, so concussions—it's not a matter of if, but when it happens."[59] High school girl soccer players get concussions at twice the rate of boys, and soccer is the number one cause of concussion among girls' sports. But boys are also at substantial risk, and parents who believe their sons are playing a low-risk, contact-free sport are often surprised to find out that

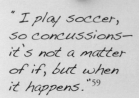

soccer concussions are common among both boys and girls. According to the Center for Injury Research and Policy, high school soccer players suffer more concussions than all baseball, softball, wrestling, and basketball players combined.

The reason for these concussions is the same as it is in adult soccer—concussions occur when a player attempts to head the ball and collides with another player, a goalpost, or the ground. However, young people are at particular risk because they have had less time to practice heading the ball and are often not taught correctly. According to former soccer player Samantha Sanderson, who cofounded Concussion Connection with Long, when a player heads the ball correctly, the arms are extended for protection. But if both players are not trained in proper form, injuries can result. "There were times where you'd get your arms out and elbow someone because they don't have their arms out and aren't doing it correctly,"[60] Sanderson explains.

Players can also get injured during practice, often due to risky drills created by well-meaning volunteer coaches. Former professional soccer player Taylor Twellman says he often sees dangerous drills in youth practice. "A parent [coach] will kick the ball in the air—a hard kick—and the kid is supposed to head it. They'll do that twenty times. I struggle to understand the thinking. One, the kid in the game is heading once or twice. Two, the ball in the game isn't going anywhere near the velocity that it is when the parent kicks it in practice."[61] Soccer balls can travel at speeds as high as 74 miles per hour (119 kph) during professional play, and a child who heads a ball improperly when it is traveling at high speed can easily sustain a concussion. In response to the dangers of heading, the American Youth Soccer Organization discourages heading for players under ten years of age. However, heading is still taught by thousands of youth soccer programs all over the country, and the organization has no plans to ban the practice.

Post-Concussion Syndrome and the Classroom

While young athletes are more at risk for concussions generally, they are also more likely to suffer from post-concussion syndrome

Depression and Post-Concussion Syndrome

When Matt Glass sustained a concussion during a high school football game, he did not report it and returned to play. Six weeks later a second concussion threw him into severe post-concussion syndrome for more than a year. Students like Glass often feel as though they have lost their identities to post-concussion syndrome, and they become so depressed that they contemplate suicide. "No one understood how it felt to have everything taken away—football, academic intelligence, even the way I felt and acted," Glass explained.

For patients like Glass, doctors sometimes prescribe drugs to alleviate some of the more severe symptoms, being careful that a medication for one symptom does not exacerbate another. For instance, an antidepressant can alleviate depression but cause either drowsiness or insomnia. A sleep aid can help a patient with insomnia, but it can also impede that patient's ability to concentrate. No medication is currently available that can help the brain heal, and it is best that only a trained neurologist prescribe medication to alleviate post-concussion syndrome symptoms.

Quoted in Robert Cantu and Mark Hyman, *Concussion and Our Kids*. New York: Houghton Mifflin Harcourt, 2012, Kindle edition.

than their adult counterparts. As it is with adults, post-concussion syndrome is often caused by a second concussion occurring before the brain has a chance to heal from the first. Symptoms vary in intensity and duration and almost always include intense headaches that can last for days at a time. Young athletes often find that their sleep is interrupted or they suffer from insomnia. Stimuli such as loud noises or the stressful environment of school can cause light-headedness or fainting. Cognitive ability can be affected; sufferers complain of feeling as though they are in a fog and are unable to think clearly. The emotions are also affected; anxiety, racing thoughts, poor impulse control, anger, and depression are common. As former high school athlete Michelle Pelton explained, "While all my classmates were involved in senior activities, I was home depressed and in constant pain, and life had become a blur."[62] Pelton was one of several student athletes who testified before a congressional panel on youth sports concussions in 2010. "Every day I endure memory loss, lack of concentration, depression, slow processing speed and cognitive effects that make my everyday life a battle,"[63] she said.

The prescription for post-concussion syndrome in youth is the same as it is for adults: Rest the brain and eliminate any activities that can be cognitively stimulating. For the student athlete, this often means no school. Crowded and chaotic hallways, brightly lit classrooms, and the stress of classroom work can tax the brain and delay recovery. Students are often prescribed quiet rest until all symptoms subside; then activities such as reading or homework can be added back gradually. Some doctors suggest that, before returning to school, students should try to complete several hours of schoolwork at home to see if any symptoms return. "The overriding theme is not to exacerbate symptoms,"[64] explains Robert Cantu.

There are no established guidelines on how long a student should rest after showing signs of post-concussion syndrome. In addition, many school administrators are not aware of how difficult the transition back to school can be for a student. To help with this, in 2013 the American Academy of Pediatrics issued "Returning to Learning" recommendations to help school administrators, doctors, and parents understand the challenges of post-concussion syndrome. The recommendations acknowledge that "each concussion is unique and may encompass a different constellation and severity of symptoms,"[65] but they offer suggestions on how schools can help ease the transition back to the classroom. For example, rest periods can be scheduled in the school nurse's office, extra time can be given to navigate crowded hallways, sunglasses can work in class to cut down on light sensitivity, and each class period—or the school day itself—can be shortened.

Unfortunately, many students do not report their concussion symptoms until they have full-blown post-concussion syndrome. Boys are notorious for underreporting concussions, but both boys and girls can lose substantial ground in school if they delay seeking medical help. Students who regularly appeared on the honor roll start earning Fs, and many fall so far behind they have to repeat a grade. "There's an epidemic of kids whose normal trajectory is permanently stunted by head injury," explains Cantu. He tells *Rolling Stone* that post-concussion syndrome can keep children out of school for a year or more. Over time, some "pass grades again and are thought of as fine, but might have been superior instead of average."[66]

Why Are Girls More Concussion Prone?

Scientists are still not sure why girls are more prone to concussions than boys. According to Dr. Dawn Comstock of the Colorado School of Public Health, "The true answer is probably a combination of reasons." She and Dr. Kevin Crutchfield, who directs the Comprehensive Sports Concussion Program at LifeBridge Health, think that because girls tend to have weaker muscles and tighter ligaments in their necks, their ability to absorb impacts is reduced. They also speculate that, because migraine headaches are so similar to post-concussive headaches, there may be a connection between women's propensity to get migraines and their susceptibility to concussions. Comstock also theorizes that hormones may play a role. Fluctuations in estrogen levels have been known to make the brain more susceptible to seizures in epileptic females, and scientists think that these changes may also make girls and women more vulnerable to concussions.

Quoted in Chelsea Janes, "Reducing the Number of Concussions in High School Girls' Soccer Is a Daunting Task," *Washington Post*, April 24, 2014. www.washingtonpost.com.

Youth Sports Organizations Take Action

The most substantial progress in reducing sports concussions has been made in youth ice hockey. Following the lead of Hockey Canada, in 2011 USA Hockey banned body checking before the age of thirteen (previously, body checking was permitted for eleven- and twelve-year-olds). The league said it intended the ban to eliminate "intimidation-type blowup hits resulting in head trauma among younger players."[67] But the ban was also meant to remove the distraction of body checking and allow players to learn fundamentals, such as how to skate well or handle a stick. One official even described the ban as "a skill development initiative."[68]

Because studies have shown that body checking is the cause of most concussions in ice hockey, it was hoped that the ban would significantly reduce concussions in the youngest hockey players. A 2013 study presented at the Fourth International Conference on Concussion in Sport confirmed this. It found that eleven- and twelve-year-old hockey players who played in leagues that allowed body checking were three times more likely to sustain concussions than those who played in leagues that did not allow body checking. The study's authors concluded that "these findings have important implications for further body checking policy change to reduce the public health burden of injury and concussion in youth ice hockey."[69]

Other sports organizations have taken smaller steps. The National Federation of State High School Associations, the organization that writes the rules for high school–level sports, held a concussion summit in 2014 to discuss how to minimize concussion risks in high school athletes. The National High School Athletic Coaches Association provided concussion education sessions during its 2014 summer convention. And in cheerleading, USA Cheer implemented a new protocol for head injury in the summer of 2014 to teach coaches and cheerleaders how to prevent, identify, and seek treatment for head injury.

Progress Made at the Local and State Level

Most of the changes aimed at reducing concussions in youth sports are made on the local and state level, either by school districts, local sports leagues, or state or local legislators. Many of these changes have been made to youth football. For instance, in an attempt to reduce the opportunity for concussions to occur during practice, Texas banned consecutive days of two-a-day football practice for high school players. A school district in Fresno, California, eliminated full-contact football practice in the off-season for the same reason. Many states have passed laws requiring concussion training for coaches and education for parents and youth. The Zackery Lystedt law, which has now been adopted by all fifty states, requires that anyone under age eighteen who is suspected of having a concussion may not return to play until he or she is cleared by a medical doctor. Nearly all states have also adopted formal return-to-play protocols, and Massachusetts even requires all youth athletes to receive a neurological baseline assessment. About four thousand high schools across the nation voluntarily take baseline assessments of their players using the computer program ImPACT, as do most large university sports programs.

Other localities are taking proactive steps to make youth sports safer in the future. Fairfax County, Virginia, is participating in a study by the Children's National Medical Center that is trying to determine if any genetic markers make an individual more concussion prone. Student athletes spit into cups so their genomes can be studied. Researchers hope to soon be able to counsel students to avoid certain sports depending on their genetic makeup. "We may actually find out, 'You know what? You're not set up to be a football player. You might be a better tennis player,'"[70] explains neuropsychologist Gerard Gioia.

Youth Football's Dilemma

The most concussion-prone youth sport is tackle football, and the largest national youth football league is Pop Warner Little Scholars—a program with more than 425,000 participants in forty-three states run largely by volunteer coaches. Pop Warner acts as a feeder program, preparing student athletes for school football programs, which usually start in middle school. In many localities, Pop Warner offers tackle football to children as young as five and as light as 35 pounds (16 kg).

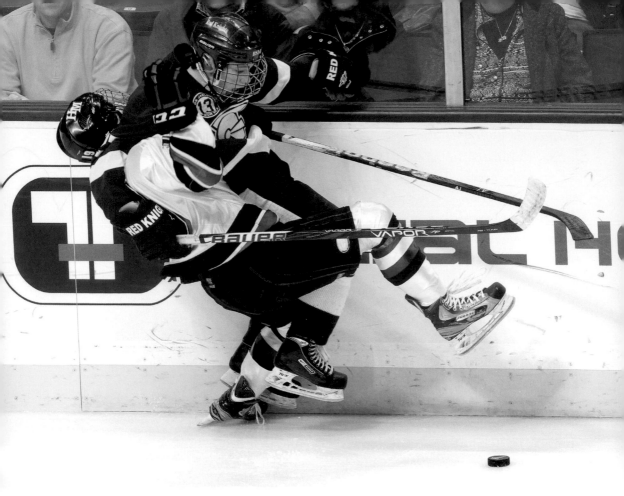

Youth players battle for the puck during a hockey game. Bans on body checking among hockey players age thirteen and younger have proved successful in reducing the frequency of concussions.

Although scientists do not have definitive proof that tackle football is too dangerous for kids, study after study indicates that this is so. A recent study found that children as young as seven years old are experiencing the same forces during hits as adults do—some higher than 80 g. In addition, studies show that the brains of young people can be changed by contact sports even if they never suffer a concussion. "I've seen serious cognitive injuries in a nine-year-old boy," says Cantu of a Pop Warner player. "He lost the ability to remember names, as well as math and vocabulary, for the better part of a year. I never felt comfortable letting him play collision sports again."[71]

However, even though participation in Pop Warner's tackle football program declined about 10 percent between 2011 and 2013, Pop Warner president Jon Butler claims that if the organization eliminated tackle for their youngest players, parents would pull their children from the league. "We've seen proposals to get rid of tackle football for kids," Butler said. "But I truly believe that if we went in that direction, 90 to 95 percent of our numbers would drop out of Pop Warner and find another way to play tackle football."[72]

Instead, Pop Warner has instituted a slew of changes to its safety rules and policies. Limits are placed on head contact and hitting in practice. Rule changes call for no full-speed head-on blocking or tackling drills in which the players line up more than 3 yards (2.7 m) apart—a rule that critics say allows volunteer coaches to simply instruct their young players to go slightly more slowly than full speed. The organization also has a training program for its volunteer coaches so that they are knowledgeable about concussions and teach proper tackling techniques. The league also proposes placing player-safety monitors at league practices and games and even installing accelerometers in helmets so that kids and their coaches do not have to decide if a hit may have caused a concussion. Brooke de Lench, founder of the youth sports website MomsTEAM, claims that accelerometers are good for everyone. Her business paid to install the devices in the helmets of her local youth football team. "The kids want the accelerometers, either in their helmet or as an earbud or a mouthpiece," de Lench says. "They want that responsibility"—of determining when they might have suffered a head injury—"taken away from themselves."[73] However, although accelerometers detect some concussions, they can hide those that occur at very low accelerations, putting more kids at risk for second-impact syndrome.

> "I've seen serious cognitive injuries in a nine-year-old boy. He lost the ability to remember names, as well as math and vocabulary, for the better part of a year."[71]
>
> — Dr. Robert Cantu.

More to Be Done

Experts believe that there is much more that can be done to reduce concussions in young athletes. Cantu proposes several simple changes in his book *Concussions and Our Kids*, such as improving the neck strength of student athletes, requiring chin straps on batting helmets, eliminating the headfirst slide in baseball, and requiring girl lacrosse players to wear helmets. But Cantu and other safety advocates feel that to make real progress in preventing concussions in young people, contact in sports should be eliminated for those younger than fourteen. This includes eliminating heading for young players in soccer and tackling for young football players. Cantu claims that at fourteen, most children are skeletally mature and their nerve fibers are fully protected by myelin. Also, at fourteen, most children are emotionally and intellectually sophisticated enough to fully understand the risks of contact sports and, with the help of their parents, make an informed decision.

Facts

- According to a 2013 poll by HBO's *Real Sports* and the Marist Institute for Public Opinion, one in three Americans said that knowing about the damage concussions can cause would make them less likely to allow their sons to play football.

- A 2013 poll by CNN found that 80 percent of the public considers concussions sustained by middle school and high school players to be a serious problem.

- The National Academy of Sciences found that high school athletes who play football, lacrosse, soccer, and baseball were more likely to experience concussions than were college-age players.

- The head is involved in more baseball injuries than any other body part. Almost half of all injuries to children in baseball involve the head, face, mouth, or eyes.

- According to the *American Journal of Sports Medicine*, boys' lacrosse accounted for the third-highest rate of concussions among all sports, after football and ice hockey.

Who Is to Blame for Concussion Risks to Athletes?

At the heart of the sports concussion debate is the question of responsibility: Who is responsible for protecting athletes from concussions? Some believe responsibility lies with the adult athletes themselves, who willingly choose to play dangerous sports. Others believe that professional sports leagues are no different than any other employer and should protect their players from the catastrophic damage concussions can cause. And still others believe society, which creates a demand for violent sports, is ultimately responsible. This debate has recently taken place against the backdrop of a lawsuit filed against the NFL. In that suit more than forty-eight hundred professional football players accused the league of deliberately misleading players about the dangers of concussions.

In youth sports the debate centers on how to balance the benefits of athletics with the risks of concussions. Some believe parents should be responsible for deciding whether or not their children take part in contact sports like football and ice hockey. Others feel that it is society's job to keep children safe and that youth and school sports leagues or the government should take steps to ensure that young athletes are not put at undue risk. The most radical of these advocates believe that children and teens should not play contact sports like football at all, regardless of the benefits.

Underlying the debate for both adult and youth athletes is the cultural meaning of sports. Sports like football are associated with distinctly American traits like physical and mental strength and determination. As Obama said in his opening remarks to the White House Healthy Kids and Safe Sports Concussion Summit, sports are "fundamental to who we are as Americans and our culture. We're competitive. We're driven. And sports teach us about teamwork and hard work and what it takes to succeed not just on the field but in life."[74] However, that attitude has created a mentality that teaches athletes to play through the pain and sacrifice their well-being for the good of the team. This has caused countless athletes to ignore concussion symptoms until their lives were destroyed by post-concussion syndrome or a neurodegenerative disease like CTE or early onset Alzheimer's.

> "Sports teach us about teamwork and hard work and what it takes to succeed not just on the field but in life."[74]
>
> — Barack Obama, forty-fourth president of the United States.

The Lawsuit Against the NFL

On June 7, 2012, more than two thousand former NFL players filed a lawsuit against the NFL, claiming that the league "exacerbated the health risk by promoting the game's violence" and "deliberately and fraudulently"[75] misled players about the potential for concussions to lead to long-term brain injuries. Over the next year, thousands more players joined the suit or filed suits of their own. In late 2013 the NFL and the players came to a no-fault settlement agreement of $765 million, to be paid out over twenty years. That agreement would provide immediate assistance to players who may not live to see the results of a protracted trial. It would also allow the NFL to avoid answering uncomfortable questions about fraud and negligence. Many thought the amount was far too low—especially since the NFL made $9.2 billion in revenues in 2012. As former offensive tackle Lincoln Kennedy said, "They want to make it go away as quickly as possible. Litigation is bad for business. . . . Basically you're throwing some crumbs out to the former players and saying, 'Hey, take this and make do with it.'"[76]

The judge agreed with this sentiment. She rejected the initial settlement offer because she doubted there would be enough money to support future claims—especially for expensive-to-treat conditions such as ALS. The NFL reconsidered and removed the $765 million upper limit on payouts, and in July 2014 the settlement was finally approved. In the lawsuit, the players had claimed that the NFL's MTBI Committee acted to deliberately mislead players of concussion risk with the series of articles it published in *Neurosurgery* and by its recommendations to the league. Because the lawsuit was settled, the question of whether or not this is true may never be answered.

Consenting Adults

The NFL lawsuit has sparked national debate about whether or not adults who are paid to play extremely dangerous sports like professional football should also be compensated for the injuries they sustain. As one online commenter writes, "I mean we get [it], football is dangerous, it gives people concussions. That's why the pros get millions of dollars to compensate for the fact that they'll be in a wheelchair by the time they're forty."[77] However, players' advocates point out that twenty years ago NFL salaries were much more modest than they are now. Few players who are now in their forties and fifties—especially linemen, who are more prone to CTE and other neurodegenerative diseases—could afford health care after they retired. Kennedy claims that he knows many retired players who cannot afford to treat their concussion symptoms. "They don't know if the reason why they're acting up on their first wife or the reason why they're so violent is because they've got something that's off in their brain due to a concussion. . . . But guys are scared to try to get evaluated because they can't afford it. It's that cut and dry. They can't afford it."[78]

Critics of the lawsuit also believe that the players' claim that they were misled by the NFL is simply untrue. Many believe that it is not possible to engage in a game where, as sports writer Buzz Bissinger puts it, "Player A wears a helmet and tries at full speed to kill Player B, also wearing a helmet and at full speed"[79] and not expect to sustain some brain injury. Bissinger goes on to assert that

"Basically you're throwing some crumbs out to the former players and saying, 'Hey, take this and make do with it.'"[76]

— Former NFL offensive tackle Lincoln Kennedy.

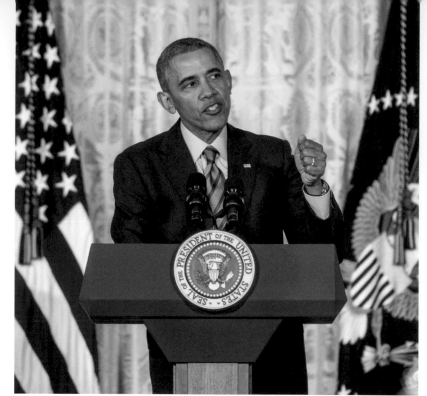

President Barack Obama addresses the White House Healthy Kids and Safe Sports Concussion Summit in May 2014. Although sports are a fundamental part of American culture, some wonder if the emphasis on competition encourages athletes to minimize concussion symptoms at great risk to themselves.

"every player in the NFL knows the possible risks down the road, whether it is Alzheimer's or the well-known realities of crippling arthritis and being able to walk only with a cane."[80] From this point of view, concussions are just one risk of many.

And although that risk may have been minimized by the NFL, a wealth of information about concussion risks has appeared in the media over the years. For instance, an article published in *Sports Illustrated* in 1994 clearly outlined the dangers of repeated head injury. In the article, Dr. James P. Kelly, director of the Brain Injury Program at the Rehabilitation Institute of Chicago, is quoted as saying, "It isn't just cataclysmic injury or death from brain injuries that should concern people. The core of the person can change from repeated blows to the head."[81] The article, titled "Doctors Warn That Repeated Concussions Can Lead to Permanent Brain Dysfunction," describes post-concussion syndrome in detail.

Desperate to Play

Although the argument that players should have known the risks has some merit, many think it is unrealistic to expect rookies fresh out of college to put their careers in jeopardy because they are concerned about the possibility of concussions causing cognitive problems later in life. Many NFL players come from poor backgrounds, and for some, football is their only way out of poverty. For instance, sixty NFL players have come out of a small region of the Florida Everglades known as Muck City, where unemployment is estimated to be higher than 40 percent. As *New York Times* reporter Bryan Mealer describes it, "The town's migrant quarter resembles something on the outskirts of Port-au-Prince, Haiti, or Kampala in Uganda. Some families have recently resorted to catching rainwater to survive because their utilities have been cut off for nonpayment."[82] In this region and others like it, football might be the only escape young men have from a future of poverty, incarceration, and early death. After making it all the way to the NFL, a player from such a background might hide concussion symptoms to avoid losing his spot on the team.

Rolling Stone commentator Matt Taibbi sees only two ways out of the concussion dilemma faced by the NFL and its players. He writes:

> Either we completely change the game, turning it into a wrap-tackling non-contact sport that'll be about as exciting as a Stay-Puft version of rugby, or else we just get all those penniless kids coming out of the SEC [Southeastern Conference] to sign waivers before they join the league. Then we'll sit back as fans and pretend that what happens to them after they retire is not a problem.[83]

Taibbi is pointing out—sarcastically—that if the game is not changed, the only solution is to force poor young men to sign away their rights to a safe workplace if they want to play in the NFL.

Giving Kids an Edge

In youth sports no one expects children or teens to be responsible for making long-term decisions about their health. The controversy is mainly among parents: those who want their children to play contact sports and those who believe the risk of concussion is too great. Parents who support contact sports believe it is im-

College Players Need Protections

Concussive and subconcussive hits that college players sustain can have devastating effects later in life. CTE has been found in football players as young as seventeen years old, and at least one college player who had never sustained a concussion also had the disease and may have committed suicide because of it. Yet college students are too old to be protected by the Zackery Lystedt law, nor do they have the level of medical support available to NFL players.

In an interview with the *New Republic*, Obama expressed his concern for college students in the concussion controversy:

> I tend to be more worried about college players than NFL players in the sense that the NFL players have a union, they're grown men, they can make some of these decisions on their own, and most of them are well-compensated for the violence they do to their bodies. You read some of these stories about college players who undergo some of these same problems with concussions and so forth and then have nothing to fall back on. That's something that I'd like to see the NCAA think about.

Quoted in Franklin Foer and Chris Hughes, "Barack Obama Is Not Pleased," *New Republic*, January 27, 2013. www.newrepublic.com.

portant to learn tackling, body checking, or heading the ball as early as possible. Girls' soccer coach Haroot Hakopian agrees. She thinks that not teaching heading to young players causes injuries later on. "The teaching of the skill, it keeps getting passed along, passed along, passed along and they get to high level high school and high level club, they haven't really practiced it," Hakopian said. "So they start doing it, they start doing it incorrectly." [84]

Some parents also believe that learning the fundamentals of a sport at an early age will give their children an advantage that may one day lead to a sports scholarship.

These parents often object when a sports league tries to limit contact in practice or during play, or when a doctor suggests taking the same precautions. "Whether it's starting kids later or doing fewer drills, we hear the same thing over and over," says Robert Cantu. "It's 'I'm not signing him up for flag football. My kid needs to learn how to tackle.'"[85] Cantu notes that many parents let their enthusiasm for their children's sports career overwhelm their instinct to protect them from injury.

However, the idea that young people will not succeed in sports unless they start early has been debunked by sports professionals. New England Patriots quarterback Tom Brady is widely thought of as one of the greatest quarterbacks of his generation, yet he did not play organized football until his freshman year of high school. In soccer, former pro player Taylor Twellman insists that nothing is lost if heading the ball is not taught until age fourteen. And the ban on body checking until thirteen in youth ice hockey has not resulted in any reduction in skill level of the young players. Cantu believes that the children who start young in contact sports may have an edge for a short time, but eventually all motivated kids will reach their own level of excellence.

Conflicted Parents Want More Education

Other parents are conflicted about whether or not to allow their children to participate in contact sports. Even Obama, who played basketball and football in school, has expressed that ambivalence. In his address at the Healthy Kids and Safe Sports Concussion Summit, he said, "I learned so many lessons playing sports that I carry on to this day, even to the presidency."[86] But he also told the *New Republic*, "If I had a son, I'd have to think long and hard before I let him play football."[87] Parents like Obama—who want their children to experience the benefits of sports without the risk of brain injury—tend to see education as a viable solution. Educating the public helps secure funding for research and to pay the salaries of athletic trainers—professionals skilled at recognizing the signs and symptoms of concussion. Only 42 percent of high schools have access to athletic trainers due to a lack of funding. Educating players will encourage them to recognize and report concussions when they happen. One study found that 66 percent of teen athletes who sustained a concussion did not feel it was serious enough to tell an adult. Teens also need to know the signs and symptoms of concussion. According to former college football player T.J. Cooney, creator of a short documentary on the dangers of concussions called *The Silent Epidemic*, "For my entire playing career, I thought extreme headaches were part of the game."[88]

Critics Resist Change

Finally, educating volunteer coaches could help make play safer for young people. However, some are concerned that volunteer coaches—many of whom learned their techniques on high school teams decades ago and have supplemented their knowledge by watching the pros—are not as open to education as they should be. According to former NFL linebacker Eddie Mason, "The coaches that coach this game . . . don't embrace change very well. . . . You can implement rules, you can implement changes, but until the football community embraces the reality of the sport, the reality of concussion, the reality of the damage that comes along with it if you start at an early age, that's the problem."[89]

There are also supporters of youth football and other contact sports who believe that the risks of concussion are grossly overstated. In his book *The War on Football*, Daniel J. Flynn argues that concussions could be reduced to almost nil with proper coaching techniques. He also claims that contact sports give boys a structured environment to do what they would be doing anyway. "In a nation where obesity, not head injuries, remains the primary children's health concern, talk of banning youth football lacks perspective. Try as we might to repeal biological laws, boys reaffirm them by fighting, wrestling, and tackling."[90] Flynn also notes that nineteen out of every twenty tackle football players in the United States are high school age or younger. Preventing these young people from

"For my entire playing career, I thought extreme headaches were part of the game."[88]

— T.J. Cooney, creator of the documentary *The Silent Epidemic*.

playing football would essentially end the sport—especially since professional leagues rely on youth programs for their players. In this Flynn might be correct. As more scientific proof of the dangers of concussions comes to light, high schools fearing lawsuits may very well drop their football programs, which will eliminate the feeder system for the pros. As one high school football coach writes, "I believe it's only a matter of time before medical research buries football under an undeniable truth: that we shouldn't be playing this game."[91]

Part of America's Culture

The reason why so many Americans find it difficult to accept that contact sports may be too dangerous to play is that sports are deeply interwoven into the fabric of the culture. For some people, sports

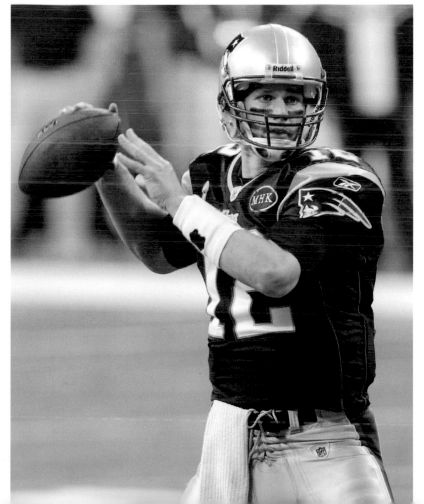

New England Patriots quarterback Tom Brady, shown here during Super Bowl XLVI in 2012, is an example of a successful professional athlete who did not begin playing sports as a young child.

give their life meaning. One such individual was Dave Coleman, a thirty-two-year-old semipro football player who was blindsided by a tackle and killed on impact during a charity football game in 2012. According to his mother, Coleman was not a happy person: He had lost jobs and relationships because of his anger, he had mismanaged his money and was struggling financially, and he had been arrested several times. "Other than his children, football was the only positive thing he had going on in his life," his mother said. "The rest of his life was just one heartbreak after another."[92]

After Coleman's death his brother Anthony (also a semipro football player) spoke about the sport. "We give our hearts, our souls to this game. This game is more than any one of us. It's more. It's football. It keeps us together through thick and thin. We put our families aside, we put everything aside, to play hard."[93] Anthony's speech implies that he felt that playing football was somehow worth the sacrifice of his brother's life—a difficult thing to understand until one realizes that Dave regularly drove two and a half hours each way to football practice, spending all of his money on gas, equipment, and fees. To the Coleman brothers, football was an opportunity to find meaning and glory in life. According to Anthony, Dave died a warrior's death, doing what he loved.

The American Warrior

The metaphor of warfare is carried over into nearly all sports. Players join together against a common enemy. They sacrifice for their brothers or sisters, pushing themselves, playing hurt, giving up opportunities to shine for the benefit of the team. As one online commenter to the Coleman story writes about football, "It's the greatest game ever. War without death! . . . Our will versus their will! At the same time the game is cerebral. Our strategy versus theirs. Who can execute better? Who is better prepared? It takes a full week to prepare for an opponent! They may be physically superior but if we execute our plan we can still defeat them! . . . GLORIOUS BATTLES!"[94] The lessons of sports revolve around the idea of teamwork and sacrifice. And this is why so many players try to play through their concussions—and will continue to do so, regardless of the amount of education they receive. If they

Football Builds Character

A high school teacher and football coach—who wishes to remain anonymous—expressed his ambivalence about football in a 2013 essay for *Sports Illustrated*. Even though he believes that football is far too dangerous and will soon fade from American life, he acknowledges how much he and his students get from the game. He writes:

> There is no denying that football is a special game, that it presents the most challenging crucible in all of sports. In the entitled suburb where I teach, there aren't many challenges. Students are adversity-deprived and lack opportunities to develop coping mechanisms to deal with the intense stress that occurs when the best laid plans in life go awry. All sports are intense in their own way, but football is different: no other sport plays just once a week; no other sport practices so many specific situations; no other sport has so many highly specialized positions; no other sport depends on 11 people being on exactly the same page on every single play. Football's lessons of teamwork, perseverance, regimen, and physical and mental toughness are more strenuous than other sports. . . . The physical and mental stress . . . ultimately produces individuals who are better tempered to deal with crisis and adversity.

Quoted in MMQB with Peter King, "A Moral Dilemma," October 24, 2013. http://mmqb.si.com.

leave the game, they let down their teammates, violating the very spirit of team sport.

There is another side to contact sports like football and ice hockey that few are willing to acknowledge. As sportswriter Kevin Van Valkenburg puts it, for some players, "there is something primal and exhilarating about delivering a blow that knocks another man off his feet. Done right, it's as pleasurable and addictive as any drug."[95] The violence of contact sports has strong appeal for fans as well. Bissinger writes, "Violence is not only embedded in football; it is the very celebration of it. It is why we like it. Take it away, continue efforts to curtail the savagery, and the game will be nothing, regardless of age or skill."[96] Many fans agree with Bissinger, which is why leagues are finding it more and more difficult to ensure player safety and still maintain a healthy bottom line. As one online commenter writes, "Football is becoming watered down and ridiculous. Watch the ratings fall as less and less big hits happen. People don't want to watch a bunch of 250 pound uneducated men run up and down a field to tag each other, they watch it for the hits."[97]

While these types of sentiments are an undeniably ugly side of contact sports, they explain why the controversy over concussions has been brewing for so many decades. In a world where concerns about safety have infiltrated nearly every aspect of daily life, neither players nor fans want to give up their last link with a more violent and dangerous world, one where hard work and sacrifice pay off and anyone can, for a brief time, be a hero. Ultimately, there may be no way that sports leagues can do enough to protect these players, who put their health at risk for the chance of glory.

"Violence is not only embedded in football; it is the very celebration of it. It is why we like it."[96]

— Sports commentator Buzz Bissinger.

Facts

- Thirty-six percent of respondents to a 2013 CNN poll said they view the NFL less favorably based on its handling of the concussion controversy.

- An ESPN survey found that about 18 percent of those polled claimed the concussion debate has made them less likely to follow football or watch it on television.

- In a survey designed to test students' knowledge and attitudes about concussions, 54 percent of respondents said they would rather win a state title game because the star player decided to play with a concussion than lose that game because the player was forced to sit out.

- According to an ESPN survey, about half of NFL fans polled believe that hard hits need to be minimized to reduce injuries, while the other half believe that hard hits are what make football a great game.

- A University of Washington study found that in girls' soccer, more than half of players who suffer concussions do not leave the game.

- A study by the University of Toronto found that mixed martial arts fighters have a higher risk of concussion than boxers or football players.

- A 2012 study in the *Clinical Journal of Sports Medicine* found that the odds of a child wearing a helmet while skiing or snowboarding was 9.55 times higher if their parent also wore a helmet.

Source Notes

Introduction: Concussions Damage the Brain

1. Quoted in Mark Fainaru-Wada and Steve Fainaru, *League of Denial*. New York: Crown, 2013, Kindle edition.
2. Quoted in Fainaru-Wada and Fainaru, *League of Denial*.
3. Quoted in Michael Farber, "The Worst Case," *Sports Illustrated*, December 19, 1994. http://sportsillustrated.cnn.com.
4. Quoted in Farber, "The Worst Case."
5. Quoted in Alan Schwarz, "NFL Acknowledges Long-Term Concussion Effects," *New York Times,* December 20, 2009. www.nytimes.com.

Chapter One: What Are the Origins of the Concussion Controversy in Sports?

6. Quoted in Michael Kirk, "The *Frontline* Interviews: Chris Nowinski," *Frontline*, June 12, 2013. www.pbs.org.
7. MacDonald Critchley, "Medical Aspects of Boxing, Particularly from a Neurological Standpoint," *British Medical Journal*, February 16, 1957, p. 359.
8. Quoted in Robert H. Boyle and Wilmer Ames, "Too Many Punches, Too Little Concern," *Sports Illustrated,* April 13, 1983. http://sportsillustrated.cnn.com.
9. Quoted in Fainaru-Wada and Fainaru, *League of Denial*.
10. Fainaru-Wada and Fainaru, *League of Denial*.
11. Quoted in Jim Gilmore, "The Frontline Interviews: Leigh Steinberg," *Frontline*, March 29, 2013. www.pbs.org.
12. Quoted in Fainaru-Wada and Fainaru, *League of Denial*.
13. Quoted in Fainaru-Wada and Fainaru, *League of Denial*.
14. Quoted in Fainaru-Wada and Fainaru, *League of Denial*.
15. Quoted in Dave Caldwell, "Pro Football's Necessary Headaches: To NFL Players, Concussions Are a Price of Playing the Game," Philly.com, October 30, 1994. http://articles.philly.com.
16. Quoted in Michael Kirk, "The *Frontline* Interviews: Dr. Ann McKee," *Frontline*, May 20, 2013. http://www.pbs.org.
17. Quoted in Bob Hohler, "Major Breakthrough in Concussion Crisis," Boston.com, January 27, 2009. www.boston.com.
18. Quoted in Alan Schwarz, "NFL Scolded over Injuries to Its Players," *New York Times,* October 28, 2009. www.nytimes.com.
19. Quoted in Schwarz, "NFL Acknowledges Long-Term Concussion Effects."
20. Quoted in Kirk, "The *Frontline* Interviews: Dr. Ann McKee."

Chapter Two: How Dangerous Are Concussions?

21. Quoted in Paul Solotaroff, "The Truth About Concussions and High School Football," *Rolling Stone,* January 31, 2013. www.rollingstone.com.
22. Robert Cantu and Mark Hyman, *Concussion and Our Kids.* New York: Houghton Mifflin Harcourt, 2012, Kindle edition.
23. Quoted in Jeffrey Kluger, "Headbanger Nation," *Time,* February 3, 2011. http://content.time.com.
24. Cantu and Hyman, *Concussion and Our Kids.*
25. Cantu and Hyman, *Concussion and Our Kids.*
26. Quoted in Jeff Z. Klein, "Study Finds Concussions in Hockey Underreported," *New York Times,* November 1, 2010. www.nytimes.com.
27. Quoted in Klein, "Study Finds Concussions in Hockey Underreported."
28. Cantu and Hyman, *Concussion and Our Kids.*
29. Quoted in Kirk, "The *Frontline* Interviews: Chris Nowinski."
30. Quoted in Samford University, "McKee Describes Tragic Consequences of Brain Trauma," October 14, 2013. http://howard.samford.edu.
31. Quoted in Helen Thompson, "Evidence Mounts Linking Head Hits to Permanent Brain Injury," NPR, December 3, 2012. www.npr.org.
32. Quoted in Loyola University Health System, "Do Sports Concussions Really Cause Chronic Traumatic Encephalopathy?," ScienceDaily, December 2, 2013. www.sciencedaily.com.
33. Quoted in Jon Solomon, "Meet Ann McKee, the Woman Who Could Save Football from Itself," AL.com, October 11, 2013. www.al.com.
34. Quoted in Solomon, "Meet Ann McKee, the Woman Who Could Save Football from Itself."
35. Quoted in Kirk, "The *Frontline* Interviews: Chris Nowinski."
36. Quoted in Mike Fish, "Rushing to Find a Connection," ESPN, November 27, 2012. http://m.espn.go.com.
37. Quoted in Solotaroff, "The Truth About Concussions and High School Football."
38. Quoted in Serena Gordon, "Football Injuries May Trigger Harmful Immune System Response," HealthDay, March 6, 2013. http://consumer.healthday.com.
39. Quoted in Gordon, "Football Injuries May Trigger Harmful Immune System Response."
40. Quoted in Steve Fainaru and Mark Fainaru-Wada, "CTE Found in Living Ex-NFL Players," ESPN Outside the Lines, January 22, 2013. http://espn.go.com.
41. Quoted in Sean Gregory, "The Problem with Football: How to Make It Safer," *Time,* January 28, 2010. http://content.time.com.

Chapter Three: Are Adult Leagues Doing Enough to Protect Players?

42. Quoted in Mark Cannizzaro, "Are NFL Kickoff Returns Dead as We Know Them?," *New York Post,* September 21, 2013. http://nypost.com.
43. Gus Turner, "The 10 Dumbest Rule Changes in NFL History," Complex Sports, September 5, 2013. www.complex.com.

44. Quoted in Judy Battista, "'Train Wreck of a Play' Collides with Consciences," *New York Times,* December 15, 2012. www.nytimes.com.

45. Quoted in NFL Head, Neck and Spine Committee and Bill Bradley, "NFL's 2013 Protocol for Players with Concussion," NFL.com, October 1, 2013. www.nfl.com.

46. Jeff Nixon, "What the NFL Still Gets Wrong About Concussions," the *Nixon Report* (blog), May 23, 2013. http://jeffnixonreport.wordpress.com.

47. Quoted in Brad Balukjian, "Hockey Still Plagued by Concussions, Despite Rule Changes," *Los Angeles Times*, July 17, 2013. www.latimes.com.

48. Quoted in Greg Wyshynski, "This Is Why NHL Concussion Protocols Fail," Yahoo! Sports, May 7, 2014. https://sports.yahoo.com.

49. Quoted in Fox News, "Football Helmets Do Little to Prevent Concussions, Study Finds," February 18, 2014. www.foxnews.com.

50. Quoted in *Huffington Post*, "Football Concussions Crisis Sparks Debate over Helmet," December 16, 2013. www.huffingtonpost.com.

51. Quoted in *Huffington Post*, "Football Concussions Crisis Sparks Debate over Helmet."

52. Quoted in Mark Derewicz, "Where G-force and Gray Matter Meet," *Endeavors*, May 14, 2008. http://endeavors.unc.edu.

53. Quoted in Derewicz, "Where G-force and Gray Matter Meet."

54. Quoted in Kirk Jenness, "Cautionary Tale for MMA: Olympic Boxing Drops Headgear, Adds 10 Pt Must Scoring," *Mixed Martial Arts News*, March 24, 2013. www.mixedmartialarts.com.

55. Matt Taibbi, "The NFL's Head Game," *Rolling Stone,* September 3, 2012. www.rollingstone.com.

Chapter Four: Are Schools and Youth Leagues Doing Enough to Protect Kids?

56. Quoted in Ken Belson, "Football's Risks Sink In, Even in Heart of Texas," *New York Times*, May 11, 2014. www.nytimes.com.

57. Quoted in Chelsea Janes, "Reducing the Number of Concussions in High School Girls' Soccer Is a Daunting Task," *Washington Post*, April 24, 2014. www.washingtonpost.com.

58. Barack Obama, "Remarks by the President at the Healthy Kids and Safe Sports Concussion Summit," White House Office of the Press Secretary, May 29, 2014. www.whitehouse.gov.

59. Quoted in Janes, "Reducing the Number of Concussions in High School Girls' Soccer Is a Daunting Task."

60. Quoted in Janes, "Reducing the Number of Concussions in High School Girls' Soccer Is a Daunting Task."

61. Quoted in Cantu and Hyman, *Concussion and Our Kids*.

62. Quoted in Alan Schwarz, "High School Athletes Detail Troubles with Concussions to a House Panel," *New York Times*, May 20, 2010. www.nytimes.com.

63. Quoted in Schwarz, "High School Athletes Detail Troubles with Concussions to a House Panel."

64. Quoted in Jan Hoffman, "Concussions and the Classroom," *New York Times*, October 27, 2013. www.nytimes.com.

65. Quoted in Hoffman, "Concussions and the Classroom."

66. Quoted in Solotaroff, "The Truth About Concussions and High School Football."

67. Quoted in Cantu and Hyman, *Concussion and Our Kids*.

68. Quoted in Cantu and Hyman, *Concussion and Our Kids*.

69. C.A. Emery et al., "Does Changing Policy to Disallow Body Checking Reduce the Risk of Concussion in 11 and 12-Year-Old Ice Hockey Players?," *British Journal of Sports Medicine*, vol. 47, no. 5, 2013. http://bjsm.bmj.com.

70. Quoted in Kluger, "Headbanger Nation."

71. Quoted in Solotaroff, "The Truth About Concussions and High School Football."

72. Quoted in Tom Farrey, "Study: Impact of Youth Head Hits Severe," ESPN Outside the Lines, February 22, 2012. http://espn.go.com.

73. Quoted in Stefan Fatsis, "Why Do We Let Kids Play Tackle Football?," *Slate*, November 14, 2012. www.slate.com.

Chapter Five: Who Is to Blame for Concussion Risks to Athletes?

74. Obama, "Remarks by the President at the Healthy Kids and Safe Sports Concussion Summit."

75. Quoted in Jim Avila, Enjoli Francis, and Lauren Pearle, "Former NFL Players File Lawsuit Against League on Concussions," ABC News, June 7, 2012. http://abcnews.go.com.

76. Quoted in Rob Trucks, "Former NFLer: 'I Know More and More Guys That Are Just Lost,'" Deadspin, January 31, 2014. http://deadspin.com.

77. Jahcorbett, August 29, 2012, comment on ESPN Video, "The Price of Playing Semi Pro Football," August 28, 2012. http://espn.go.com.

78. Quoted in Trucks, "Former NFLer."

79. Buzz Bissinger, "NFL Playoffs: Why Football Needs Violence," Daily Beast, January 17, 2011. www.thedailybeast.com.

80. Bissinger, "NFL Playoffs."

81. Quoted in Farber, "The Worst Case."

82. Bryan Mealer, "The Way Out," *New York Times*, February 2, 2013. www.nytimes.com.

83. Taibbi, "The NFL's Head Game."

84. Quoted in Janes, "Reducing the Number of Concussions in High School Girls' Soccer Is a Daunting Task."

85. Quoted in Solotaroff, "The Truth About Concussions and High School Football."

86. Obama, "Remarks by the President at the Healthy Kids and Safe Sports Concussion Summit."

87. Quoted in Franklin Foer and Chris Hughes, "Barack Obama Is Not Pleased," *New Republic*, January 27, 2013. www.newrepublic.com.

88. Quoted in Cantu and Hyman, *Concussion and Our Kids*.

89. Quoted in Fatsis, "Why Do We Let Kids Play Tackle Football?"

90. Daniel J. Flynn, *The War on Football: Saving America's Game.* Washington, DC: Regnery, 2013, Kindle edition.

91. Quoted in MMQB with Peter King, "A Moral Dilemma," October 24, 2013. http://mmqb.si.com.

92. Quoted in Kevin Van Valkenburg, "Games of Chance," ESPN, December 19, 2012. www.espn.com.

93. Anthony Coleman, "The Price of Playing Semi-Pro Football," ESPN Video, August 28, 2012. http://espn.go.com.

94. Masternameless34, August 29, 2012, comment on ESPN Video, "The Price of Playing Semi-Pro Football," August 28, 2012. http://espn.go.com.

95. Van Valkenburg, "Games of Chance."

96. Bissinger, "NFL Playoffs."

97. Teamfive, August 29, 2012, comment on ESPN Video, "The Price of Playing Semi-Pro Football," August 28, 2012. http://espn.go.com.

Related Organizations and Websites

Barrow Resource for Acquired Injury to the Nervous System (BRAINS) Program

Barrow Neurological Institute
350 W. Thomas Rd.
Phoenix, AZ 85013
phone: (602) 406-6281
website: www.thebarrow.org/
Neurological_Services/B.R.A.I.N.S._Program

The BRAINS Program at St. Joseph's Hospital and Medical Center is a treatment and rehabilitation center for victims of traumatic brain and spinal cord injury. Its website has links to concussion videos, special reports, and general information about concussions.

Brain Injury Research Institute (BIRI)

5309 Landing Ln.
Moon Township, PA 15108
phone: (888) 542-3152
website: www.protectthebrain.org

The BIRI is a research institute founded by Dr. Julian Bailes and Dr. Bennet Omalu, the doctors who first discovered and researched CTE in the brain of deceased football player Michael Webster. The website provides information on CTE, dementia pugilistica, mild traumatic brain injuries, and concussions, as well as links to current research.

BU Center for the Study of Traumatic Encephalopathy (CSTE)

Boston University School of Medicine
72 E. Concord St.
Robinson Complex, Suite 7380
Boston, MA 02118
phone: (617) 638-6143
e-mail: cbaugh@bu.edu
website: www.bu.edu/cte

The CSTE was created as an independent academic research center for the study of CTE. The CSTE website contains information about the CSTE brain bank, as well as details about past and current research studies.

Centers for Disease Control and Prevention (CDC)

1600 Clifton Rd.
Atlanta, GA 30333
phone: (800) 232-4636
website: www.cdc.gov/concussion/HeadsUp/online_training.html

The CDC provides information on prevention and control of concussion and traumatic brain injury on its website, including reports and fact sheets, data and statistics, and a link to its free online concussion training program for coaches, Heads Up: Concussion in Youth Sports.

Concussion Inc.

e-mail: info@muchnick.net
website: http://concussioninc.net

Concussion Inc. is a website created by sportswriter Irvin Muchnick. The website features a collection of Muchnick's articles that help spread information about traumatic brain injury and CTE among athletes, including the stories of Chris Benoit and Dave Duerson.

ConcussionWise

website: www.concussionwise.com

ConcussionWise offers online concussion education courses on prevention, response, and recovery of concussion. Courses are free for athletes, parents, and coaches.

Sports Concussions

Brain Injury Alliance of New Jersey
825 Georges Rd., 2nd Floor
North Brunswick, NJ 08902
phone: (732) 745-0200
e-mail: info@bianj.org
website: www.sportsconcussion.com

Sports Concussions is a website created by the Brain Injury Alliance of New Jersey. The website contains information aimed at youth sports participants, parents, coaches, and educators, including a list of online resources and publications.

Sports Legacy Institute (SLI)

230 Second Ave., Suite 200
Waltham, MA 02451
phone: (781) 819-5706
e-mail: info@sportslegacy.com
website: http://sportslegacy.org

The SLI is dedicated to solving the concussion crisis by advancing the study, treatment, and prevention of concussion and related brain trauma through advocacy, education, policy development, and medical research. Its website contains a wealth of educational and advocacy information.

ThinkTaylor

350 Granite St., Suite 1102
Braintree, MA 02184-4999
e-mail: info@thinktaylor.org
website: http://thinktaylor.org

ThinkTaylor is an education and advocacy organization dedicated to changing the culture surrounding sports concussions. It was founded by Taylor Twellman, a Major League Soccer all-star who retired in 2010 due to complications from multiple concussions.

Additional Reading

Books

Robert Cantu and Mark Hyman, *Concussions and Our Kids*. New York: Harcourt, 2012. Kindle edition.

Linda Carroll and David Rosner, *The Concussion Crisis: Anatomy of a Silent Epidemic*. New York: Simon and Schuster, 2011.

Mark Fainaru-Wada and Steve Fainaru, *League of Denial*. New York: Random House, 2013.

Daniel J. Flynn, *The War on Football: Saving America's Game*. Washington, DC: Regency, 2013.

Christopher Nowinski, *Head Games*. Oakbrook Terrace, IL: Head Games the Film, 2014. Kindle edition.

Bennet Omalu, *Play Hard, Die Young: Football Dementia, Depression, and Death*. Lodi, CA: Neo-Forenxis, 2008.

Periodicals

Ta-Nehisi Coates, "The NFL's Response to Brain Trauma: A Brief History," *Atlantic*, January 25, 2013.

Jan Hoffman, "Concussions and the Classroom," *New York Times*, October 27, 2013.

Jeffrey Kluger, "Headbanger Nation," *Time*, February 3, 2011.

Paul Solotaroff, "The Truth About Concussions and High School Football," *Rolling Stone*, January 31, 2013.

Documentaries

League of Denial: The NFL's Concussion Crisis. *Frontline*. Directed by Michael Kirk, aired October 8, 2013. www.pbs.org/wgbh/pages/frontline/sports/league-of-denial/credits-51.

Head Games: The Global Concussion Crisis. Directed by Steve James. New York: Variance Films, 2012. http://headgamesthefilm.com.

Internet Sources

Paul McCrory et al., "Consensus Statement on Concussion in Sport—the 4th International Conference on Concussion in Sport Held in Zurich, November 2012," *Clinical Journal of Sports Medicine*, March 2013. http://journals.lww.com/cjsportsmed/Fulltext/2013/03000/Consensus_Statement_on_Concussion_in_Sport_the_4th.1.aspx.

NFL Head, Neck and Spine Committee, "NFL Head, Neck and Spine Committee's Protocols Regarding Diagnosis and Management of Concussion," NFL.com, October 1, 2013. http://static.nfl.com/static/content/public/photo/2013/10/01/0ap2000000254002.pdf.

Websites

The Concussion Blog (http://theconcussionblog.com). *The Concussion Blog* is a rich source of current information and perspectives on the concussion controversy. The blog's author, certified athletic trainer Dustin Fink, states that he supports prevention and management of concussions but is against reducing contact in sports.

League of Denial: The NFL Concussion Crisis (www.pbs.org/wgbh/pages/frontline/league-of-denial). *Frontline*'s web page devoted to the 2013 documentary *League of Denial* contains a wealth of information about concussions, including a full-length documentary, in-depth interviews, articles, and Concussion Watch, a project that tracks officially reported head injuries in the NFL.

NFL Concussion Litigation (http://nflconcussionlitigation.com). *NFL Concussion Litigation* is a blog published by attorney Paul D. Anderson, an export on concussion law. The blog is devoted to the recent concussion lawsuits by players against the NFL and contains news and scholarly articles, court documents, and analysis.

Real Clear Sports (http://realclearsports.com). Real Clear Sports is a website devoted to aggregating sports news and commentary. It has links to more than fifty articles dealing with concussions in sports from multiple perspectives, including concussion safety and sports preservation.

Index

Note: Boldface page numbers indicate illustrations.

Aiello, Greg, 9, 24
Aikman, Troy, 14–15
Ali, Muhammad, 12–13, 25
Alzheimer's disease, 8, 16, **22**, 33
    among former NFL players *vs.*
        general population, 25
American Academy of Pediatrics, 60
American Journal of Sports Medicine,
    39, 66
amyotrophic lateral sclerosis (ALS,
    Lou Gehrig's disease), 8, 25, 53
Apuzzo, Michael, 17–18, 19
athlete(s)
    college, lack of protection for, 72
    have incentives to hide injuries,
        44–45
    as warrior, 76–78
    youth, dilemma for parents of,
        71–74
axons, 28, **30**
    protective covering of, 29–30

Bailes, Julian, 30, 38
Barr, Bill, 15
baseball
    head injuries in, 66
    prevalence of catchers experiencing
        concussion symptoms in, 39
    prevalence of concussions in, 53
Bazarian, Jeffrey, 37–38
Bellucci, Victoria, 55
Benoit, Chris, 20
Bissinger, Buzz, 69–70, 78
blood-brain barrier, 37–38
boxing, 12–13, 50

    amateur, ban on headgear in, 51
    force of punch in, 25
    steps taken to reduce concussions
        by, 51–52
Bradshaw, Terry, 6
Brady, Tom, 73, **75**
brain
    developing, vulnerability of, 29–30
    second-impact syndrome and, 33
    subconcussive blows and damage
        to, 34–35, 49
    tau protein tangles in, 16–17,
        33–34
Brain Research Institute, 10
British Journal of Sports Medicine, 51
Brown, Melik, 48
Butler, Charles, 51
Butler, Jon, 64–65

Cantu, Robert, 32, 34, 37, 46, 60,
    64
    on evaluating head injuries, 31
    on myelin coating of nerve cells,
        29–30
    on parents' objections to safety
        reforms, 73
    on reforms needed to prevent
        concussions, 65–66
Carpenter, Dan, 41
Carson, Harry, 6
Casson, Ira, 12–13
Center for the Study of Traumatic
    Encephalopathy, 21, 37
Centers for Disease Control and
    Prevention, 8
cheerleading, 56, **57**, 62
chronic traumatic encephalopathy
    (CTE), 7–8, 33–35

deaths related to, 19–20, 24, 53
dispute over causes over, 22–23,
  35–37
recognition of, 12
Clinical Journal of Sports Medicine,
  10, 79
Coleman, Anthony, 76
Coleman, Dave, 76
Comstock, Dawn, 61
concussions, **27**
  among girls, 56
  as cause of CTE, dispute over,
    35–37
  causes of, 27–28
  children's vulnerability to, 28–30
  definition of, 26
  educating public on dangers of,
    8–9
  g-forces and, 48
  linear/rotational forces causing, 29
  prevalence of, 8, 10
  recent breakthroughs in, 37–38
  recovery from, 31–32
  symptoms of, 30–31
  in youth sports, White House
    summit on, 55–56
Concussions and Our Kids (Cantu), 65
Condi, Frank, 45–46
Conte, Stan, 39
Cooney, T.J., 74
Cotto, Miguel, **13**
Critchley, MacDonald, 12
Crutchfield, Kevin, 61
CTE. *See* chronic traumatic
  encephalopathy

deaths, related to chronic traumatic
  encephalopathy, 19–20, 24, 53
de Lench, Brooke, 65
dementia pugilistica (punch-drunk
  syndrome), 12–13
depression
  post-concussion syndrome and, 59
  suicide and, 35
DETECT Study (Center for
  the Study of Traumatic
  Encephalopathy), 37

Ditka, Mike, 46
Duerson, Dave, 24

Easterling, Ray, 24
Echlin, Paul, 31

Fainaru, Steve, 14
Fainaru-Wada, Mark, 14
Flynn, Daniel J., 74–75
football
  as character builder, 77
  force of impact on lineman during
    typical play in, 39
  objections to rule changes in,
    41–42, 74–75, 78
  youth, 63–65
    decline in enrollment in, 9
    parents' conflicts over, 54–55,
      71–74
  See also National Football League
Fourth International Conference on
  Concussion in Sport, 35, 62
Frazier, Joe, 25
Freel, Ryan, 24
Frontline (TV program), 14, 22, 24,
  32, 36–37

Gehrig, Lou, 25
g-force, 48
Glass, Matt, 59
Goodell, Roger, 23–24, 41
Grange, Patrick, 53
Guskiewicz, Kevin, 18, 46–48

Hakopian, Haroot, 72
Hamilton, Ronald, 16–17
Head Games (Nowinski), 21
head guards
  ban on, in amateur boxing, 51
  for soccer players, 50
Head Impact Telemetry (HIT)
  system, 47–48
Healthy Kids and Safe Sports
  Concussion Summit, 55–56
helmets
  accelerometers/sensors in, 46–48,
    65

as ineffective in preventing concussions, 45–46

high school football players, percentage reporting concussions, 10

Hoge, Merril, 6, 14

horse racing, amateur, concussion rates in, 39

ice hockey, 39
  prevalence of concussions in, 31
  youth, ban on body checking in, 62
  See also National Hockey League

Immediate Post-Concussion Assessment and Cognitive Testing (ImPACT) program, 42

Injury Surveillance System (National Collegiate Athletic Association), 53

International Amateur Boxing Association, 51

Karantzoulis, Stella, 35

Kelly, James P., 70

Kennedy, Lincoln, 68, 69

kickoff returns, 41

lacrosse, 56, 65–66

Long, Lauren, 57, 58

Long, Terry, 19

Lou Gehrig's disease. *See* amyotrophic lateral sclerosis

Lovell, Mark, 14

Malanga, Gerard, 18

Maroon, Joseph, 13–14, 17

martial arts fighters, 79

Martinez, Sergio, **13**

Mason, Eddie, 74

McCain, John, 50–51

McElroy, Greg, 45

McHale, Tom, 22–23

McKee, Ann, 21, 22–23, 24, 34, 38
  on children's vulnerability to concussions, 29
  on chronic traumatic encephalopathy, 35–36

Mealer, Bryan, 71

Mild Traumatic Brain Injury (MTBI) Committee, 8, 15
  subpar research by, 17–19

Moore, Matt, 54–55

myelin, 29–30

NASCAR, 39

National Academy of Sciences, 66

National Basketball Association (NBA), prevalence of concussions in, 53

National Collegiate Athletic Association (NCAA), 41

National Federation of State High School Associations, 62

National Football League (NFL)
  denial of problem with concussions by, 11–12
  desperation of athletes to play in, 70–71
  lawsuit against, 68–69
  prevalence of concussions in, 53
  steps taken to reduce concussions by, 9, 40–41
  criticism of, 41–42, 74–75, 78

National Hockey League (NHL), 44, 45

Neurosurgery (journal), 8, 17–19, 69

neurotransmitters, 28, **30**

New Republic (magazine), 72, 73

NFL Head, Neck and Spine Committee, 23–24, 42

Nixon, Jeff, 44

Nowinski, Chris, 11–12, **20**, 20–21, 32–33, 36–37

Obama, Barack, 56, 68, **70**, 73
  on concussions in college athletes, 72

Omalu, Bennet, 15–17, 19, 21, 38

opinion polls. *See* surveys

Parkinson's disease, 8, 25

Paterno, Joe, 46

Pellman, Elliot, 8, 15

Pelton, Michelle, 60

Plummer, Gary, 16
polls. *See* surveys
Pop Warner Little Scholars, 63–65
post-concussion syndrome, 8–9,
    32–33
    depression and, 59
    in young athletes, 58–61
Professional Fighters Brain Health
    Study (Cleveland Clinic), 51
punch-drunk syndrome (dementia
    pugilistica), 12

Ramirez, Ainissa, 46
Randolph, Christopher, 35
Return to Play guidelines, 32, **34**
Robinson, Sugar Ray, 25
Rolling Stone (magazine), 61

Sanderson, Samantha, 58
S100B protein, 37–38
Schwarz, Alan, 21
Seau, Junior, 24
second-impact syndrome (SIS), 33,
    56, 65
The Silent Epidemic (documentary),
    74
Smith, Alex, 44–45
soccer
    concussion in girls and, 57
    heading the ball in, 48–50, **49**
Sports Concussion Institute, 39
Sports Illustrated (magazine), 12–13,
    70, 77
Sports Legacy Institute, 21, 39
Steinberg, Leigh, 14–15, 16
Stern, Robert, 24
Stiles, Nathan, 33, 34
Strzelczyk, Justin, 19
subconcussive blows, 34–35
    in boxing, 52
    chronic traumatic encephalopathy
        and, 23, 72
    in football/ice hockey, 39
    in soccer, 49
suicide(s), 24
    associated with chronic traumatic

encephalopathy, 19–20, 35
    depression and, 35, 59
surveys
    on attitudes toward NFL/football,
        79
    of pro baseball catchers on
        experiencing concussion
        symptoms, 39
    on youth sports concussions as
        serious problem, 66
symptoms
    of chronic traumatic
        encephalopathy, 35
    of concussion, 30–31
        prevalence of baseball catchers
            hit by foul balls experiencing,
            39
    percentage of athletes not
        experiencing, after concussive
        blow, 39
    of post-concussion syndrome,
        32–33

Tagliabue, Paul, 15, 23
Taibbi, Matt, 52, 71
tau protein, 16–17, 33–34
    in diagnosis of CTE, 35, 37, 38
    tangle of, **22**
Thomas, Owen, 34
Turner, Gus, 41–42
Twellman, Taylor, 47, 58, 73

University of Pittsburgh Medical
    Center, 10

Van Valkenburg, Kevin, 77–78

The War on Football (Flynn), 74
Washington Post (newspaper), 55
Waters, Andre, 19
Webster, Michael "Iron Mike," 6–7,
    7, 15–16, 19
Wisniewski, James, **43**, 45

Zackery Lystedt law, 63, 72

Picture Credits

Maury Aaseng: 27, 34

© John A. Angelillo/Corbis: 75

AP Images: 7, 57, 64

© Brian Cahn/ZUMA Press/Corbis: 20

Ken Cendeno/Corbis: 70

Thomas Deerinck, NCMIR/Science Source: 22

© Frank Franklin II/AP/Corbis: 13

Francois Paquet-Durand/Science Source: 30

© Howard C. Smith/ISI/Corbis: 49

© Paul Vernon/AP/Corbis: 43

About the Author

Christine Wilcox writes fiction and nonfiction for young adults and adults. She has worked as an editor, an instructional designer, and a writing instructor. She lives in Richmond, Virginia, with her husband, David, and her son, Doug.